Behind My Heart

Finding Life's Voice Over There

CAROL ULRICH

A Loncar Ink Book

BEHIND MY HEART

Contact Information:

carol_ulrich@hotmail.com

ISBN 978-0-9970939-0-2

DEDICATION

To those who can no longer compete with their human strength but stay in the ring anyway.

Maybe they choose to stay because they understand that God is their real strength, providing not just the will, but also the means to get up over and over. Maybe that's why some get up and others don't. Some call upon God, and others forget His name. Maybe that's why everyone roots for the underdog. They cheer for him because they know that if he can find strength greater than his human capacity—God—at that moment, even what looks like a loss is really the greatest victory. And sometimes when the odds are beat and the impossible is achieved, letting the less than become more than enough to win, everyone applauds and rejoices. Not because of the score but from the unspoken knowing of everyone watching the fight: that God was there and He was the reason for the victory.

Table of Contents

Acknowledgments 1

Introduction 2

Here And Over There 6

Part 1: The Fall 10

Part 2: Flying Further Into My Descent 33

Part 3: Thrashing In The Chasm 53

Part 4: Choosing Life 68

Part 5: Learning My Truth 104

Part 6: The Rise 134

Part 7: Beautiful Truth 223

Acknowledgments

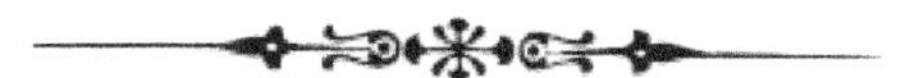

I was blessed to make it across the finish line and I now bow my head to acknowledge the others who ran valiantly alongside of me for as long as they could. I also want to acknowledge and cheer for my sisters and brothers that are still trying to complete their journey and are, perhaps, searching for breath.

I thank everyone I met and everything I experienced on my cancer journey that moved me closer to my destination, my Truth in God. My bridge back home to peace was built with a bunch of dust, cancer gods, chemicals, tears, prayers, family, friends, broken pieces of me, airplanes, strangers, limos, a minivan, a pontoon, angels, country songs, blinding snow, and God's love. A hodge podge of people, circumstances, and experiences filled me with love, faith, and joy. I humbly assembled and moved across my bridge one Truth at a time. It was not created as a temporary passageway. It was constructed strong, steady, and beautiful enough so that I would always remember what's on the other side. Acknowledging the brilliant collage of people and events through this story is what will keep it brightly lit so that I will find my way back to the Truth of *Over There* every time I slip away.

Introduction

I knew my story was going to include God—I had no idea God was my story.

I sat righteously right between religion and spirituality when I was diagnosed with breast cancer. I had judgments about both and the way each approached the subject of God. I had painfully and adamantly defended my feelings for forty-seven years. But during my chemo treatments, when I almost died and I met God, it didn't matter what I believed or what those who thought differently believed. I wasn't in a church or an ashram; I was in the backseat of my minivan, dying. I was only with God. That is when I found out that God is there for everyone, regardless of what they think they believe.

This story shares my journey to find and stay connected to God and cure my cancer. Yes, this is a story about cancer, but it's also a story about how, in any given moment, you can choose life. Cancer revealed to me that I could no longer live a life where my mind inflicted constant hidden pain in my heart. I had to sit with my cancer in the shadow of my mind's pain and hurt until I found another way to live. And I did, I miraculously found the 'Truth of Life', but only after I became physically and mentally unable to participate in the world I had created *Here*.

There was no one more disconnected from what was going on in my subconscious mind than me. I had no idea that I had a negative, stressful whisper in my ear all day every day telling me I wasn't good enough. Telling me in order to not be a *less than* I always had to try harder and do more. I didn't know that this voice cast an unseen shadow over all my happiness and accomplishments. I had no idea that it was this unknown thinking that stressed my immune system, leaving me open to getting cancer and then leaving me unable to heal my cancer.

As a child, I grew up in a traditional middle class family with a blue collar dad that loved our family very much and was home every night for dinner and a stay-at-home mom that took great care of my sisters and me. I was in Girl Scouts and had a paper route. My days included: summer camp, slumber parties, and track meets. I made friends easily, was mischievous, and laughed a lot. As a standout athlete, I received a scholarship to play basketball in college. After graduating with academic honors from college, I went on to law school and passed the bar exam. As an adult, I found career success in higher education and technology sales earning a very nice living. I bought my first home in my twenties, traveled to many places around the world, and eventually married a wonderful man and had loving children. I'm not saying that I didn't have ups and downs along the way or that life didn't require a lot of hard work, because it did, but on the whole I believed I was happy and was grateful for my good fortune. My well-crafted picture of a perfect life and easy smile masked my stressful subconscious thinking, until cancer stripped me of my façade.

It doesn't matter that I was wrong about how I subconsciously saw things, felt things, and then believed them. It doesn't matter that these were the same thoughts, emotions, and beliefs I formed as a child. They were the way I operated in the world. By the time I got cancer, my heart had been under attack for over forty years. I was used to the pain; it felt normal. I broke because I did not love myself enough to find a way to acknowledge the pain, let alone stop it. You should not have to break to love someone, especially yourself.

In order to heal my broken heart and rise from my hidden pain, I had to turn around and begin looking to a place I had forgotten: *Over There*. I found *Over There* only after I escaped my subconscious *less than* mind *Here*. *Over There* is where I would cure my cancer. *Over There* is the most sacred place inside of me. The place of my Truth. The place of God. I found my healing through the peace of God—but not the judgmental God I had heard about in Sunday school. The God I have come to know brought me unfathomable love that made me realize I was already more than enough. Please accept this story as an offer of my Truth to you—Truth as I experienced it.

I learned that everyone has a choice as to when they look *Over There*. The choice is not *how*. *When* is the only choice you need to make. Ask and you shall receive, not with a magic pill or potion, but with the most unpredictable and astonishing messengers of Truth and beacons of light along the way.

Although the journey is sacred, the journey itself is not the goal; the goal is to find your way back to the peace of your Truth in God so you can move into the blessings only God can bestow. God will always be there waiting until you are ready to hear His voice. He loves you just as you stand in this moment. He has no judgments, only unconditional love and forgiveness anytime you ask. At any moment you can choose to seek Him– and in that moment you can find and know Him.

At the time, I thought breast cancer was my worst nightmare. Now it represents a sacred moment in time that led me back to God. My understandings about Truth and God are blessed gifts now instilled in my heart. They occurred during my illness in seemingly benign moments, passing thoughts, random experiences, and sometimes utter horror. I was too sick or too tired to acknowledge many of these revelations as they were occurring. Some caught me by surprise, and I could not find an explanation for them at the moment. Others scared me, and I didn't know what to do with them so I pushed them away. I miraculously held on to a few, knowing they could only have been from God. As I look back and piece them all together, the design and layering is breathtaking. They were perfectly woven into a beautiful blanket of God's Truth—my Truth. This is how I know God was there. This is how I can show you the Truth of God, as I was and am: incapable of creating this beautiful portrait alone.

Here And Over There

Truth is worth acknowledgment; sometimes even tears in reverence to it. This simple Truth, when understood, will change your life. Right now, your soul or spirit is residing in a human body. You, the soul or spirit, always has been and always will be a part of God, and that makes you more than enough just as you are. Humanness by its very nature is separate and imperfect, and can even be unloving, but the part of you that is a part of God is of perfect light and love.

When I used to live exclusively *Here*, I resided in a world where all I understood was about being *less than*. *Here*, is experienced from a one-dimensional human experience where your human mind tells you that you are *less than* and separate from everyone else. The only thing inclusive about *Here* is that everyone thinks they are *less than* someone else, making them primarily concerned with their *less than* selves. People of the right age are better than people of another age. However, once someone's right age becomes another age, they too are *less than*. Similarly, even if someone is the right age but hasn't accomplished certain achievements, they are already *less than*. Correspondingly, even if someone is the right age and has attained certain achievements, they can still be *less than* other people of the right age who have greater achievements. Once you are *less than* for having turned another age or for not having better achievements, you might try to work even harder to be more. Despite your best efforts, the laws of judgment *Here* emphatically dictate that you will never be enough. You are required to judge and compare yourself to others as you try to overcome your *less thans*, and will be judged by others so that they can try to overcome their *less thans*. The hard truth of *Here* is that even if you are the right age, with the best of achievements, and you live in the perfect part of *Here*, in the perfect house, with granite counter tops, you will still know that you are *less than*—because of your job, your body, your significant other, your car, your finances, your education, your kids, your friends, your shoes, or someone's judgments about you. This leaves you trapped *Here*, in a solitary place of unrelenting judgment.

Here is a tough place; it does not permit peace. There is never enough, and you are never enough. *Here* only recognizes and rewards the winners at its made up games. It's a place that says a number on a man-made scoreboard makes someone else *less than*. It puts the need to be better before balance, profits before parenting, pushing through before health, power before peace, and love of others finds itself a distant second to lust of everything else. And those running *Here* want you to either believe God is not real or He is out to harshly judge you for being a *less than* sinner just like they do.

The law of judgment is a thick cloud of smoke that hangs in the air, choking off your singular self-worth every day. Love in the world of *Here* is tenuous and mostly conditional. Joy is fleeting because you think you are not worthy of it. Hope is then secretly squandered so that you can continue to think that at some point you will be *more than*.

This leaves you with only fear to hold on to; fear of knowing that you will always be alone and never enough. So everyone tiptoes around *Here*, hiding, being *less than* in their designer shoes that cripple their calloused feet and squeeze their broken hearts.

Now, I know there is a world *Over There* with God that yields only abundance, a world where everyone always feels included. No one ever questions whether they are good enough, because *Over There* everyone knows there is no such thing as *less than*. *Over There* is illuminated so you can see everything differently. Life is viewed only through your heart. *Over There* is a world where there is no such thing as judgment, only love.

Who wouldn't want to live where you are more than enough, even as you stand barefooted? Where your kids can be themselves, you can happily drive your old car, and you like your job? Where peace prevails? After all, location, location, location is where we all want to live, right? The problem for developers *Here* is that anyone can live *Over There*. So they blow thick smoke around *Here* to stop you from finding *Over There*—precisely calculating that people will not be able to clear their minds and catch their breath long enough to rise above the haze of *Here* and understand that there is somewhere else: a place *Over There*, where we can choose to live anytime we open our hearts to God.

My unfolding and embracing of life and Truth, which I later came to call God, was not spontaneous. This story covers eighteen months of my life following my breast cancer diagnosis. In the beginning of my journey, I thought I had fallen down into my *less than* chasm due to my cancer diagnosis. I came to realize I had created the darkness long before the cancer showed up. Cancer is what forced me to acknowledge and sit in the desolate vacuum that had been hollowed out by my mind *Here* and that separated me from God *Over There.* The chasm is neither *Here* nor *Over There*; it is the absence of light in between. This is the space reserved for choice: the choice for understanding and the choice for healing.

Some people cross that void with ease, most through pain. I chose the latter, agonizingly unaware that I was making that choice. I believed there was only one place to go once outside of the valley of *less than* error, back to the only world I had known: *Here*, in front of my heart. *Here* is where I could indulge in the familiar pain from my *less than* mind over healing my heart and crossing the emptiness to find the unknown: *Over There.*

It took me almost too long to leave the nowhereness of my *less than* spiritual limbo and secure my footing in the place that I forgot so that I could save my life. I needed to find my Truth to understand why my mind kept punching my heart. As I sat in my *less than* chasm behind my heart, time lovingly wrapped its arms around me and held me in gentle stillness, silencing my mind, allowing me to hear the voice of life. You learn from behind your heart that time is timeless and that there is always another tomorrow and another choice for life.

PART 1

The Fall

The roller coaster of emotions was straight up, straight down, full circles, dark tunnels, holding my breath, grasping too tightly, almost slipping out of my seat and plunging to my death, throwing up, screaming, laughing, then having no fear and raising my hands in the air. In the end the ride stopped, I got off and collected my picture of that snapshot in time.

In 2012, we were now living in North Dakota. As I was finishing up my gynecological examination, a friendly nurse mentioned that I was coming due for a mammogram and she would set up the appointment if I wanted her to. I told her, "It's fine to schedule it, but I'm not really worried about rushing to get one." I easily said, "I somehow know that breast cancer is not going to be the thing that takes me out." Confirming those words by adding, "Cancer is really not my thing." I went on, saying, "You know how you just know things? Well, I just know *that*." She agreed about knowing things. I then assuredly added, "If I'm going to go, it would most likely be a heart attack. That sounds more like my end game, but not cancer." Shortly after that, I had the mammogram done. It confirmed the words that had so easily fallen from my mouth.

Fourteen months after that mammogram, I found a cyst. I'd had many before, but this one was in my breast. I went to my first-line medical doctor, Dr. Internet, and read that breast cancer is not painful. Dr. Internet's words appeased my mind since the side of my right breast next to my arm was red and hurting. I had felt cysts on my body before, and they had felt exactly like this one: full of fluid, moveable, and painful. I made an appointment to get it drained. One week later the local surgeon, who had removed other cysts from my body, began the procedure of inserting a needle into my latest cyst. He hit a hard spot and a look of concern crossed his face. He said, "It doesn't feel right. It's hard." I replied in confusion, "What? I felt it last week and it was soft. How does it get hard in a week?" He replied, "Well, normally I would be really worried, but with your history of cysts it might not be anything." *Yeah, yeah, I'll go with that*, I thought. *How could it be cancer anyway? Cancer is not my thing.* The needle's contents were sent off for a biopsy. I set up an appointment to return the following Monday for the results.

That Sunday, as I was waking up, I immediately gasped to take in an extra gulp of air to catch my breath. *Odd*, I thought. *Maybe I had a scary dream.* Later that morning I was in the kitchen cooking our usual big Sunday breakfast when my husband Dan walked behind me and asked why I was breathing so hard. I told him that I didn't know but that it had already happened several times that morning. For the rest of the day, I just could not catch my breath. I had just recovered from bronchitis but didn't remember having this much trouble getting air.

Although it seemed a little odd, I had things to do and decided it was annoying but it wasn't going to kill me. Therefore, I assumed it would eventually stop, which it did… many months later.

The following day began as a usual Monday, working from home full-time in software sales and full-time as a mom. I made the kids breakfast, checked emails, got the kids off to school, had conference calls, worked on a proposal, and kept running to the cupboard to get enough M&Ms to keep going. I had forgotten about my follow-up appointment with the doctor until Dan came home from work and reminded me. I told him I didn't want to go to my appointment, thinking it was a waste of time. I had had at least six biopsies from cysts before; always nothing. Dan said I should go anyway and asked if I wanted him to come with me. I agreed to go but told him to stay home because "cancer is not my thing."

At the doctor's office, I was taken to a small room where I sat down on an uncomfortably hard chair. My seat was in the corner squeezed precisely between the wall that held the door and a wall that placed me squarely against a tiny bare desk. As I tried to get comfortable, I realized that my right arm was being poked by the light switch next to the door. The nurse informed me that I would be meeting with a physician's assistant since my surgeon was out of town. As the doctor's substitute entered the room, he nonchalantly greeted me and then proceeded to open a folder. He handed me the single piece of paper that the folder contained. The first words that jumped off the page, in bolder print than the others, were "Ductal adenocarcinoma." The carcinoma part did not sound good.

I asked, "What does this mean? Is it cancer?" As my mouth was speaking those words, my eyes were intently searching for the word "benign." I did not expect to simultaneously hear the word, "Yes" from the doctor's stand-in and see the word "malignant" jumping off the page, connecting a one-two punch to my face. I felt my head snap back from the blows and began seeing a black shadow slowly swirling around, the word "What?" echoing inside my head. It rolled around and around until it started spinning. *Wait! What? WHAT?* What kind of cancer? How much? How bad? He had no ideas and no answers. I could not even come up with good questions since I didn't know anything about cancer. All I knew was what I saw on television, and those stories never ended well. I usually changed the channel before the person died. The one thing that I did know about cancer was that I never wanted to have it.

The doctor's understudy tried looking up the diagnosis terminology in a big, thick medical book that he took from his overfilled bookcase to better explain my situation, but he could not find any answers in there either. Strangely enough, for all the thoughts I could have had as he flipped through numerous pages in the ridiculously large book, I thought, *Boy, when people on television get cancer, the news seems to be delivered much better than this.* I just sat there staring intently at the report on the otherwise bare desk, the doctor's replacement in his comfortable chair, and the big book, which held lots of words but no answers, in his fumbling hands. I sat there as calm as possible waiting for him to do something, and doing my part to not turn off the light switch. All the while I was thinking that there was some medical procedure he was trained to do after injecting my heart with this news. I assumed that he would thoroughly explain this information so it would not be so awful. I moved on to hoping he would just tell me something to have this make more sense. Then I decided I would settle for just hearing that I was going to be all right, that it was not as bad as it seemed. My last silent plea was for him to just touch my hand and say he was sorry. I wanted him to do something, *anything* to make me feel better. He did not. It was the first of many times to come that the medical community would give me a shot of pain and not even offer me so much as a Band-Aid to cover the needle site.

As he shut his gigantic, answerless book, I wanted to scream, "I have Blue Cross and Blue Shield. I deserve better than this!" My mind demanded more details. I silently screamed, *I need details!* I think I was in as much shock from hearing the news as I was at how bad the delivery of the news was being handled. I thought, "*You don't tell someone they have cancer and leave that big death-knell word sitting on a small empty desk without details. You don't send me home holding a virtual casualty report with the only detail in it being cancer. That's too scary. I need those words translated into something that I can understand so I can find a way to fix it. I can't fix what I don't know. I deserve a better meeting than this. Every day at work people demand better meetings than this from me and I deliver!*"

That was the beginning of a long series of disappointments; of learning that cancer is open-ended and scary and that no one would ever have any better answers than I had just received. Cancer was too big to wrap my human mind around.

Apparently the staff had already discussed—hopefully less awkwardly among themselves than with me—what they needed to do next, as they were busy booking more appointments for me. So I was asked to wait in the narrow hallway. Maybe they knew, as I did, that this news was too big to stay in that small room. Or maybe they knew if I flinched as I sat there, wedged between the light switch and the doctor's bare desk, I would be sitting in the dark. As I exited the room, I somehow became fixated on my age and my sons' ages and kept thinking over and over, '*I am only forty-seven and my boys are only ten and seven! I am only forty-seven and my boys are only ten and seven! I am only forty-seven and my boys are only ten and seven!*' The word "what" dissolved into a dull, black shadow of fear and was now in a continuous loop, warping through my thoughts and emotions in slow motion.

My choices, once outside the room, were turning left toward an emergency exit door or moving straight ahead toward a dim stairway that led to a dark, vacant floor below. I chose to lean on the stair rail and look into the darkened nothingness in front of me, wanting to throw up. However, I was too numb and shocked to feel my body. I didn't know what to do with myself. I just stared down into the shadows at the bottom of the stairs, becoming more anxious with every second that passed. I began to fear my mind's slow-motion reeling, as it was beginning to fixate on the blinding darkness below. Unconsciously I found my mom's name in my phone contacts. I hit the green call button not even realizing what I had done until she answered the phone.

As she said, "Hello," my reply was, "I have breast cancer." The first time you say those words it feels surreal, like you are a bad actor insincerely and awkwardly delivering your line in a way that makes the audience murmur. I felt like I was repeating hurtful gossip about myself that wasn't true. It was too soon to share what I had just been told. I should have held on to it longer, but instead I treated it like a hot potato that I needed to pass on to someone else before it exploded. This was pretty much the way I always treated myself: something to be given away, not held.

The irony of my setting was lost on me at that moment, but I was apparently staring down into the dark chasm my *less than* mind had created. I went home not knowing how to tell my husband. *I was wrong, so wrong. I'm a disappointment. I'm weak and I'm deeply flawed. I have cancer*! Now I knew why I couldn't catch my breath the day before. I wasn't sure if I would be able to find it again.

I could have fallen into the dark, vacant abyss and into a heroic coma as a military hero hurt in the line of duty, or from a skydiving accident while attempting to help someone open their chute, or even from being sickened while trying to save lives in a small, impoverished village on the other side of the world. But I didn't. I was just a forty-seven-year-old working mom using all my strength just trying to be good enough. The truth is it did not really matter. What I experienced in the shadowy void that day was formed long before that moment. It just happened to be cancer that revealed the heaping mess my mind had created. Cancer became a crude tool that I had to use to help me find my way out. The gaping pit of the chasm between me and God allowed cancer to become big enough and scary enough to send me so out of control that it handily changed all things in my life—but not before it almost took everything. There I was, now lying in the desolate and barren space of the *less than* chasm behind my heart.

My casual words to the nurse that day about not worrying about breast cancer because "it wasn't going to take me out" would haunt me every time I sank deeper into the dim gorge and closer to death. It shook the foundation of what I thought I knew about myself. My intuition now had a big red X over it and a cancer tumor beneath it. I scolded myself: "How can you ever trust anything you think again? How can you listen and trust your intuition to fight breast cancer when it told you it wouldn't take you out in the first place?" My trustworthy inner knowing of things now vaporized and I was totally engrossed in my unworthiness, my *less than.* Those words about cancer not taking me out that fell so easily out of my mouth haunted the limited vocabulary of my mind most of the time I was in treatment.

As I lay on the floor, I wasn't a non-believer, non-believer, but I wasn't a believer, believer either. Either way I felt that God was something outside of me, and that left me ultimately alone.

I had walked through life like a divine tourist using a souvenir, knock-off map that took me from wandering to lost. Over the years here and there I would dabble with trying to answer my questions about God: questions that had lingered since my childhood experiences with an intolerant priest and Sunday school stories that made me believe getting into heaven was harder than a camel passing through the eye of a needle. All I knew was I did not want to be one of the poor masses that my textbooks in college told me religion was used to control. I also did not want to be one of the *less thans* and sinners that religion was always trying to save. And the last place I wanted to be was with self-righteous religious types, the people who used God to look down at me and pronounce me as *less than* with their vehement insistence that if I didn't believe exactly what they believed, I was going to be judged, found wanting, and sent straight to hell. So I started my career, eventually got married, had kids, and left all those questions and thoughts on a shelf for later.

After giving up on religion, I pivoted toward spirituality, still hoping to find God whom I started calling the Universe. Although religion left me disappointed with God, the Universe remained unblemished in my eyes. I started reading books about spirituality, searching for clues in their secretly coded karmic messages. It was like playing a game of Battleship. I ended up with more misses than hits. Every once in a while when I thought I was getting an inkling of what they were talking about, the phone would ring and it would be my boss wanting to know when my next sale was coming in; or I would have to respond to an e-mail, meet with my son's teacher, go to the store, pay the bills, find a new phone plan, argue with a customer-service person about something, or deal with yet another remodeling project for our house. The beautiful picture for which I secretly yearned remained pieces of a puzzle that I did not take enough time to connect. I was caught up in the all-encompassing vortex of my life: getting up tired, running all day, and going to bed exhausted. As I spiraled around and around in my self-created tornado, I hit a point when I became so dizzy that I forgot it could be any other way.

When that happens you cannot even remember that tornados aren't safe, so you continue to twirl until one day at 4:10 in the afternoon it suddenly spits you out. You are then thrown across the room and hit the wall that holds the perfectly displayed snapshots of your life confined within fragile glass picture frames. At the moment of impact, they shatter spewing glass shards in every direction, leaving you and everyone and everything around you a bloodied mess. Most of the cuts appear to be just beneath the surface, so you naively think you can stand up, unable to conceive that you have been gravely wounded by superficial shards. Who knew all those years of printed perfection right in front of me, hiding my fear of not being enough, hung there already having cut me to pieces?

Through tears of desperation, trying to get my bearings, I only knew two things. My thoughts about cancer and God were like two bullet points in one of my work PowerPoint presentations. They were simple and straightforward.

- I don't know anything thing about cancer except it is big and scary and I have no idea how to fix myself.
- In a last-ditch effort, if I am in real trouble, I will hope that God is real and that He is not too busy to help me.

Regarding bullet point number one, I was way behind the power curve of understanding how cancer worked, how it was treated, and didn't think many people actually survived it. I had never watched anyone go though cancer treatment and my nativity made everything uncertain, exaggerated and surreal opening me up to a side of fear that I had never experienced.

To expand on bullet point number two, as a believer/non-believer I never actually prayed to God. Even if I was thinking from the believer side, I did not believe God wanted to hear all my petty requests. I presumed people with more pressing concerns needed Him more than I, so I honorably left Him alone. At the time, I did not realize that He is infinitely available to everyone, nor did I understand that there is no miracle too big or too small to request. I thought you had to get on a prioritized waiting list for help, like at the emergency room. A couple of times, when something more important was at stake, in order to not waste too much of His time on me, I would mostly tell God what I was doing and what He needed to do. Back then, my believer self would not describe my actions as praying so as not to upset my non-believer self. Maybe I was saving up my prayer minutes, continuing to roll them over for now.

After my cancer diagnosis, I let loose on the prayers, knowing I now had something on the "I'm in real trouble" list. I crossed my fingers, hoping God was real so He could save my life. First I pleaded for my life and then I moved on to begging for my life. When neither seemed to work, I sank even deeper down the *less than* chasm. I guess I was waiting for a text, or smoke signals, or something to confirm that my request had been granted. Now I know that my pleas to be cured may have been answered the instant I asked. Back then, I didn't understand that just because you don't see the miracle the moment you ask doesn't mean it hasn't already happened.

I now know there is a place Over There, behind my heart, where my moment begins. You can go there when it is easy, wait until life falls apart, or stumble into it, like I did, when you are about to die.

"Jesus said unto him, Thou shalt love the Lord thy God with all thy heart, and with all thy soul, and with all thy mind." Matthew 22:37

I now wonder why I never heard about how to live my life *Here* through the loving light and love of God found *Over There*. I had heard about God as a child, but He was in heaven and I was *Here*. I think on Sundays He might have been at church with us, but I was never too clear on that. At church, I mostly winced as I watched God's middleman, my priest, standing at his pulpit judging sin and feeling like he was condemning me. As an adult, I heard about spirituality, the law of attraction, and living in the moment. These brokers of a non-committal godlike entity acted much nicer when promoting their chants that alluded to a generic *Over There*. Yet most of their messages were dressed up in fancy buzzwords or clever phrases that made me feel like they came out of plastic fortune cookies. Being in sales myself, I had a hard time swallowing them.

Over There is a natural, simple, beautiful place of God's love inside of us. As I wondered around *Here* the radiance of that love became contorted and convoluted for me by a handful of religions and overmarketed spirituality gurus. Their views and actions made God an inaccessible myth to me. It wasn't just the religious dogma or the spiritual semantics that had me lost and twisted my mind around *Here*. It was also the deceptive messages that the world *Here* was advertising to me and my mind was shouting at me: there is never enough, and I would never be enough.

All this noise made me feel that I was unqualified and unworthy of finding and being in a peaceful place within myself where God resides. Once you know there is an *Over There*, nothing is more natural than living from there. Once you again find *Over There*, you will know that everyone is capable of finding it and is good enough to be there.

Before cancer, I lived my life exclusively *Here.* As I look back on my memories, I now see all the times God revealed Himself to me and I can't believe I continued to think there was only *Here.* God was jumping up and down with a neon sign over His head pointing to *Over There* throughout my life. Even though I sometimes acknowledged His brilliance, I still never saw the real light. I would look at *Over There* as if it was a fireworks show. After the bright lights faded, I would be right back *Here* with only a fading memory of His glow. The inertia of *Here* keeps you moving in a straight line at blinding speed, making any change in direction elusive. Your designer-labeled blinders block out the Truth from *Over There*, and you continue looking straight down the path of the only world you know: *Here.* If I'd known then what I know now, all I would have had to do was escape my mind *Here*, leaving my heart free to find *Over There.* Then I could have embraced what I had forgotten.

I like to think that if someone had simply told me about *Over There*, and that it was inside of me all along, then I wouldn't have had to look for help every place else first. I wouldn't have been wandering around *Here* believing that a middleman was more capable of saving me and showing me how to find my Truth than my own heart. I would have known that Truth is God. The place of your Truth is the place of God, and it can only be uncovered when you drop everything else that is not of love from your mind and heart. Through clearness and stillness, your Truth is revealed. Truth is experienced through the pure sacredness of love, nothing else. I wish I would have found the part of myself that is a part of God sooner, and not have held on to my pain almost too long.

You will see what a messy human I was and still can be. You will witness how divine crumbs of destiny and beacons of hope arrived miraculously, and how I grabbed hold of God's hand in those moments, but didn't know I was supposed to hold on. I just didn't know *how* to hold on. I did not know there was a place behind my heart, outside of my mind's thoughts of being *less than*, to sit with God—a place where I could go anytime, any day for however long I chose. I thought there was only *Here* in front of my heart but found the most beautiful place *Over There* behind my heart: a place that is with God. I learned that I could be with God every minute of every day. I could carry Him in my heart *Here* and find His love, safety, and peace *Over There*. I could move back and forth between the physical world *Here* and the Heaven of *Over There* in an instant.

My blinders were carefully crafted by my mind to fit precisely so that I was only able to see myself through my illusion of success, allowing the burden of the hurt, screaming inside of me every minute of every day, to be silenced by my mind's chaos.

The day after I received the sparse report on my cancer diagnosis, I received the important detail I had silently screamed for. Less than twenty-four hours after leaving the doctor's office, I heard what caused my cancer diagnosis, and what needed to be fixed. However, the noise in my mind was now too loud, as I sat shrieking from inside the chasm.

It was just a single thought which bothered me the second it arose, but I was unable to understand what it was telling me. I knew it was a strange thought to have, but a small part of me believed it anyway. At best what I thought was a footnote of my journey contained much of the Truth of why I got cancer and why my story went the way it did. I can still remember every detail of this simple passing thought.

I had rushed out of the house and jumped into my minivan on autopilot, not thinking about anything other than trying to get to my sons' school to pick them up on time. Since I was late, I had to park a street farther away from the school than I usually did and I could see all the other parents in their cars parked in front of me. After I stopped the minivan, and as I was moving the gearshift to park, I thought, "*Now they are all going to think that they are better than me because I have breast cancer.*" I could not believe I thought that. It felt pathetic as I reran the words for a second and third time in my head, wondering why I would think something like that. I shuddered from having had such a thought, but had to turn away from my feelings as the kids opened the doors and entered the car filled with their excitement of being out of school for the day. I had to put that awful thought away for later, just like everything else I had been thinking and feeling since my cancer diagnosis.

I now realize the power of the word "cancer." My subconscious thoughts of not being good enough slipped out into full view in my conscious mind that day. Because the day after you are told that you have cancer, you cannot lift your automatic subconscious shield of your *more thans* as a defense against the subconscious thoughts of your *less thans*. The protective shield of my achievements was not strong enough to defend me against my cancer failure. That day I could not push the subconscious thought of not being good enough down before it hit the surface by subconsciously yelling back about my education, my paycheck, or my granite countertops.

I'm not good enough… It hung there in my mind and I heard it for the first time: a subconscious thought I'd had probably a million times before, but one from which I had always been able to protect myself from hearing by subconsciously lifting my *more than* shield. Now it revealed itself. At the time, I only knew it was an off thought. I was still unaware that underneath my sureness, success, and friendly smile, I felt that way all the time. It was many months later that I caught onto this way of thinking, and could recognize it for what it was. But until then I could not forget that thought. It always bothered me, and I always wondered why I would think such a hurtful thing.

Looking back now, I see so many times when life's voice clearly told me the way out of my hurt, but I was too distracted by the noise in my mind, always trapped in its chaos and not able to hear God. My self-imposed world *Here* was run by a lying tyrant in my mind always putting me down and separating me from God. I had created a deep gash of hurt on the inside, while appearing shiny, lucky, self-confident, and happy on the outside. I thought I had it all: a loving husband, great kids, loyal friends, an outstanding education, a high-paying job, and all the other accolades of success. I thought I was living the dream. What was really going on in my subconscious mind, though, was the non-stop avoidance of again feeling the hurt of a seven-year-old girl who thought that she was not *good enough* to be accepted.

Cancer did not teach me fear; it revealed all my human fears. Through cancer, I learned how to become fearless as I lay in the warmth and protection of the hand of God. God's love feels safer than being inside a circle, yet too immense to be contained in one.

I could not find a way to shake the fear. I couldn't even stop crying after I was out of tears. I trembled until I passed out from exhaustion. I talked and talked and talked, trying to expel cancer from my body. I became nauseous and sick with a fever within days of my diagnosis. I thought I could wear fear out. I thought it would run its course. However, fear, like cancer, mutates and finds new ways to envelop the host. I told my mind over and over to quiet itself, which only caused the noise to intensify. The harder I tried to push fear out of my thoughts, the more manic the swirling became.

Early on, my friend Judy suggested that I write down some healing mantras. I know my sayings were not perfect spiritual textbook prose, but at the time they were the best I could come up with, and in the early days of cancer they were all I had to hold on to. I wrote them down using a blue permanent marker on three white index cards.

I wrote, "I have nothing to fear. I will respond to treatments with amazing results. Once the cancer is gone, it will not return. I WILL BE A CANCER SURVIVOR! I will be physically here on earth with my family and I will love them and take care of them for the next thirty-five years! I will not allow my children to suffer the pain of growing up without me in their lives. I will not leave Dan. I am healthy and happy. I will let go and trust in God. I will think positive. I ask for this or something better."

When fear was piercing through every space in my body and my mind was running like a paranoid rat on crack, I would read those cards word for word, over and over and over. I kept them in my pocket during the day and under my pillow at night. I used those words as a shield of protection from my mind so they could speak for me when I was unable to think about any words other than *cancer* and *death*.

Although cancer treatment didn't heal my tumor, it showed me that healing my heart, which heals all, is done through something unimaginable: the healing power of God.

"Put on the whole armor of God, that ye may be able to stand against the wiles of the devil…Above all, taking the shield of faith, wherewith ye shall be able to quench all the fiery darts of the wicked." Ephesians 6:11, 16

"Keep thy heart with diligence; for out of it are the issues of life." Proverbs 4:23

As my fear and tumor continued to grow, so did a new set of self-preserving behaviors and feelings that had never previously surfaced in me. One that showed up almost immediately after the word *cancer* did was a tangible sense of a bulletproof object attached to my chest over my heart. It felt real. I could picture what it looked like in my mind and somehow felt it occupying the space in front of my heart. It was rectangular, three-quarters of an inch thick, opaque, and covered most of my heart. I thought it was positioned over the middle part of my heart because that is where I was most vulnerable. My new heart guard was as real to me as the hair on my head—and thankfully stayed longer.

I did not know why it was there but guessed that maybe my heart needed protection from the relentless assault of fear. I did not dwell on the new object covering my heart because I thought I had bigger concerns about what was in my breast. However, I did start to notice that this device slowed down the automatic incoming shrapnel people hurled toward me: people who would choose to cry in front of me about my cancer; or people who told me their friend had died from breast cancer; or people who were being mean to me unaware of my cancer.

I began to notice that what used to sting my heart was now being repelled by this opaque barrier. *Weird*, I thought, *but I'll take it.* Everyone's all-access pass to hurt my feelings had been revoked. Although strange, it happened before starting chemo, so I know I was not completely out of my mind at that point, and I know it was real enough to work. Somehow a part of me had enough life-preserving instincts to grow this mechanism to block more hurt from a heart that already had too much. It was many months later that I figured out why it had come: the part of me that wanted to live knew I had to stop hurting my heart.

This is why I must tell this story, because I was running through what I called life, like most people, until I realized that the shadow inside my chasm was running me. The things that happened to me and for me came as divine crumbs, sprinkled from the Universe, miraculously taking me back to God. They nourished me until I could again find the life that I had lost.

At first I hated the tumor and would not touch my breast. When I thought about how it ruined my life and became angry with it, the lump would start to throb. I would then get even madder at it for throbbing, and the ache would further intensify. I began to notice the angry exchange of pain between my mind and my cancer. When I would hurl my emotional hurt at the tumor, I would then physically feel my mind's distress inside my breast. My psychological tactic did not lessen the stress in my mind but added additional agony to the growth in my breast. I somehow doubled my pain. So, being great at sales and a professional at causing myself suffering, I had somehow created a twofer sale on my pain: keep the upset you're trying to give away and take on the same hurt somewhere else for free. Only a top-performing go-getter like me could masterfully find a way to plunge the knife of pain twice.

I would learn in my Truth that this is a universal law; everything you give you receive, good or bad, but not today. Today I would hold back my natural instinct to touch the cancer in order to soothe our mutual pain because today my mind only wanted to punish both of us. This went on for a little over a week. Then one night before I went to bed, again agonizing over my lump, the throbbing began again. However, this time I felt sorry that I was taking my mental hurt and giving it to the growth as physical harm. I started to care about how my mind was wounding my body. I touched my breast where the cancer hid and said, "I'm not mad at you. I now know you are the only one who understands my mind's pain in the exact same way as I do. I'm scared of you and I think at this point you are afraid of me too. But who are we kidding; you are a part of me and I am the reason you are here. I'm sorry. I am really sorry for not giving us enough love, and for allowing us too much hurt. We are going to have to figure this out together. I am going to make it okay for you to go. I don't know how, but I want you to know we are on the same team. I know I need to stop allowing my mind to injure you so you can leave my body." My lump stopped throbbing when I stopped being mad at it, however I was still relentlessly mad at myself. At that point, I still did not realize that my mind wasn't just hurting my tumor; it was also pummeling my heart.

PART 2

Flying Further Into My Descent

While I was in shock and knee-deep in anxiety, I did not realize that my fear and I had been quickly herded into the corral with other cancer sheep. Inside the fence, I lived as a cancer sheep. Now that I was confined and the only thing I saw was other sheep I began to think I was one. Every once in a while when I would gaze outside the enclosure, a quick thought would pass that maybe I'm not a cancer sheep, but I knew that everyone else now saw me as a cancer sheep. Being sheep-minded now, I had to let it go. Everyone, including the cancer sheep, knows the only way cancer sheep get to leave is when a wolf drags them away for a shearing or the slaughter. I did not know that it would take a wolf in white sheep's clothing dragging me out of the corral, to find out who I really was again.

I thought I could secure my future through finding treatment outside of North Dakota. My Blue Cross and Blue Shield did come in handy for that. I found a cancer hospital in Chicago. I discovered them in the middle of the night when I could not sleep and was feverishly searching the Internet for healing answers. I didn't find those answers, but I did find a number I could call and someone was available to talk with me at 3:00 a.m. They were nice and they were very sure they knew better than anyone how to save my life. So my husband and I got our tickets to begin our descent.

When you fly to the cancer hospital, they meet you at the airport. As Dan and I collected our two large suitcases off the baggage carousel, we found the hospital's driver. As he looked at our luggage, he said, "This must be your first visit. Everyone brings big bags their first time." I did not know what that meant, but it sounded odd. The swirling in my mind now made almost everything sound strange and feel off. Things that people said kept feeling like they should have an ominous, foreboding, "Dant-dant-da!" after them. Since the driver was really friendly as he said those words, though, I smiled as if I understood his point. Later I figured out that everyone brings full bags containing everything that makes them who they are in this world for their first visit to the cancer hospital. By the time you depart, you are sheared of everything other than your cancer.

We followed the driver outside from the baggage claim area. He directed us toward a limo parked a few steps from the terminal and right alongside a McDonald's delivery truck. I said, "Wow, who knew I would have to get cancer to be a rock star." Only in my twisted heroic-coma dreams would a limo pick you up to deliver you to your cancer treatment. We settled into the far back seat looking forward. Three other rock stars and their assistants sat facing us and surrounding our view. As the car began to move, everyone started talking. As veterans of the cancer tour, they all sang freely about their cancer. The ever-amiable driver even chimed into tell us about *his* cancer. I, at this point, a little less than three weeks into my cancer, was still embarrassed that I had cancer. I did not want to be me, let alone them, so I sat quietly and tried not to cry. Then someone nonchalantly asked me what type of cancer I had. With the spotlight on me, I hesitantly said, "Breast cancer." I had only admitted those words a handful of times, and they still stung like telling a lie as they crossed my lips. Simultaneously, along with the spilling of those two words from my mouth, I could feel a wave of water filling my eyes. I was glad the lighting was low in the limo because when you continue to hold back the tide you intermittently have to release big drops of saltwater out of your portals. In the past few weeks I had learned that if I leaned forward just enough, I could make the crest of the wave fall directly from my eyes and hit my lap. This way no one would have to know I was crying except my wet jeans and my broken heart. I did this for the next forty-five minutes of the tour as I listened to the other musicians' lyrics.

It was explained to us that the cancer hospital utilized many hotels and that our hotel was the furthest from the hospital. The ever-smiling driver told us our hotel is where all the newcomers and their big suitcases stayed. At first I wondered why the new recruits stayed so far away from the hospital. A few months later I decided they place you there because it's easier to believe in the magic show when you are not sitting too close to the stage. We then checked in and fell unconscious. I was still hoping I would wake up from the heroic-coma dream that I had fallen into while performing a fearless act so I could slide right back into my life as a hero.

The next morning, we found out that in the light of day, rock stars lose their fame—today we had to ride in the tour bus. So we boarded the cancer shuttle to the hospital with the other regular musicians. As Dan and I were driven to our first-day orientation, we learned that even when you are traveling coach to the show, you are still supposed to be on stage and act happy. You need to sing songs and act perky in front of other players on the shuttle ride. We decided to be divas and mostly sat quietly unless prodded into niceties by the driver.

I had made a hundred-and-eighty-degree turn from the wave of tears the night before, and had on my winning corporate game face. I decided to have this day run like a business meeting. I had a long winning streak at those. My husband and I had agreed prior to our arrival in Chicago that we would not make any rash decisions or do any chemo on this trip. We were going to find out as much as we could and carefully weigh all our options about how to save my life; doing so on our terms, not anyone else's. I had my list of questions and knew how to consult and negotiate any deal. We ended up short selling of our objective. By the time we left the only thing we actually learned, through painful infusion, was the non-negotiable business of chemotherapy.

I stepped off the shuttle with my usual quick pace, putting my fresh face forward along with my bouncy, full head of blonde hair and, of course, my winning personality and smile. I was going to have several well-timed key meetings with the team I read about online, design a project plan, get my assigned tasks, and be on my way.

Errrr. This is the part where you hear the record scratch. My illusion that got me through breakfast and the shuttle ride without tears changed the moment I walked through the front doors of the cancer hospital. As I entered a beautiful atrium with floor-to-ceiling windows, real trees and comfortable reclining chairs, my heroic-coma dream was abruptly flooded amid a sea of people turning it into a nightmare. Today there was standing room only as everyone was checking in for their appointments. The lines to register were so long I felt like I was at Disneyland. However, it had more of a carnival feel. People of all shapes, sizes, and colors. Young and old, rich and poor. The reality hit me like a wave of heat during the summer in Las Vegas: heat that evaporates the sweat right off your face before you even know it is there. I became overwhelmed and unable to move. I just stood there, like one of those birds that keep continuously scanning their environment, looking back and forth, then back again to see if anything is different, desperate to somehow reinterpret where I was, and to feel safe again.

Through the waves of cancer, I saw snapshots of the sickest people who were so frail and gaunt that they resembled prisoners from Nazi concentration camps. They were either reclined in their chairs sleeping, or sitting and staring blankly into the beautiful space of the atrium. To have so much cancer surrounding me overwhelmed my senses and shook me to my core. Even with all the crying and everything I feared about cancer, now, seeing real people with actual cancer made me realize that what I naively thought about my frightening diagnosis was the G-rated preview of a very scary show.

Then my eyes fixated on a gaunt woman in a wheelchair by the elevators. She had a blue-and-white scarf on her bald head. It was hard to tell if she was forty or seventy. She was bent over in her wheelchair, staring down at the ground, unable to hold her torso up. I shivered and thought to myself, *She's going to die*, again hearing, "*Dant-dant-da!*" I held tighter to my husband's arm and desperately whispered, "Don't ever let that happen to me," not really believing that even in the worst version of this nightmare that would be the fate of the woman standing in *my* shoes. Even though I had been scared of everything I didn't even know about cancer, I never considered that you could be so sick that you would be doubled over and too weak to sit up in a wheelchair. The image of this poor woman haunted me from that moment on. The saying, "You don't know what you don't know" was meant for that moment. I had never considered that there was a middle part of cancer treatment. My mind always jumped from the diagnosis to the survivor's luncheon or funeral. I was not prepared for what was in between.

So I signed in and was handed my badge to wear. Printed next to my name on the badge was the capital letter P put in parentheses (P) for patient, to remind me and everyone else that I was one who had been branded. They then secured an all-day ride pass paid for by Blue Cross and Blue Shield around my wrist. Next, I was given my printed schedule, which had been set prior to my arrival. The cancer hospital's goal was to put me at ease with my new life. Everyone in the magical kingdom was friendly and upbeat. The first day ran like freshmen orientation. They earnestly try to make the most distressing thing that has probably ever happened in your life seem cheerful and normal. This well-intentioned charade not only looked awkward but also felt unpleasantly unnerving.

After witnessing the barrage of wounded soldiers in the lobby, I was now orientated to feel like I needed to join forces with the cancer-fighting team. I therefore tried to forge a tenuous bond at the welcome speech, on the tour, with the financial counselor, during the intake examination, and while getting blood tests. That was seemingly benign enough stuff I recognized from my past life. But what happens as you are embraced and led through the corridors of the hospital and then squeezed into tight machines for scans, the exercise that welcomes you to your future with enveloping arms mixes with your ever-present fear of right now. This makes your diagnosis and distress feel permanent, completely numbing your senses. This unyielding merger of emotions puts you on a scary one-way-only path. As you are pressed between the smiles and treatment schedule, the now narrow view eliminates your ability to turn around. This is how you are quickly herded into the corral with the other cancer sheep.

Looking back, I now know it had to unfold just as it did because of just how I was. Who better to fix me than me? Who better to make this plan than the subconscious mind of mine that knew what buttons to push and what pieces to move at what time for a checkmate? I was actually fighting myself; I sensed it even as I was doing it but I did not know any other way.

When I heard about the particular characteristics of triple-negative breast cancer, my first thought was, *Wow, it sounds a lot like me.* The description said that only about fifteen percent of breast cancers are triple-negative. It is aggressive and grows fast, which leaves it more vulnerable to chemo than other breast cancers. However, it quickly outsmarts the chemo and mutates. There are currently no effective chemo regimens once that happens. Even if you are initially lucky enough to have the chemo work, there are no follow-up medications to resist its return like other breast cancers. This means it reoccurs more often than other breast cancers and its aggressiveness will most likely take your life in less than a year when it does. It is one of the least known about and one of the most deadly breast cancers. With the first twenty-four months after diagnosis the most likely timeframe for reoccurrence.

Okay— unconventional, fast paced, smart, feisty, take-no-prisoners cancer. Just like me! My second thought, as bad as it sounds, was, *Well, I don't have the patience to worry about cancer coming back for the next twenty years anyway. I'm glad that I only have to think about this for the next two years and it will be over.* Knowing my cancer's traits and characteristics not only fueled my fear but my aggression toward treating it. All I kept hearing was, "Tick-tock, tick-tock."

That is how the battle lines were drawn for this most epic self-confrontation of my lifetime. I naively thought I would have an advantage since my cancer was like me—but fighting the mirror version of yourself is more futile than it appears. After unsuccessfully trying to fend off the attack of cancer, I came to realize that the most harmful weapons against you disguise themselves as the best parts of you. I seriously underestimated my strength's ability to wound me. When you are wrestling with yourself for your life, you need to find your perceived strength's "mirror opposite" to unravel the secret code that lies within you. I was crusading for whom I thought I was, and with the only strengths I had known, until I learned that what I was fighting with and what I was fighting for were actually the *problems*, not the solutions.

I thought my experience of living in the world I had created Here taught me to see around corners. I thought I knew how to navigate through this life, until I careened off the road in a near-fatal accident. I now find it ill-timed that the news only reports what happens at the exact moment an accident occurs. You never hear what happens as people are fighting for their lives. This lifesaving information is usually left unknown. I wonder why journalists don't recognize that the aftermath is the real story. That's what people need to hear: the whys and hows of the people who were hurt and survived, so they can learn the secrets of how to pick up their own wrecked self and live, maybe for the first time. Somehow

life's sacred secrets are revealed to those closest to death; to those who choose to find life through them.

Since arriving in Chicago, I had to listen to my husband Dan tell me over and over how exhausted he was, tell me the bed in our hotel room was too uncomfortable and he could not sleep. That's why he was tired. He just needed to rest. This was coming from a man who since I met him over a decade earlier could not sit still and was always doing something. My cancer diagnosis turned him into a man who was now unable to get out of bed. I didn't know what to do. What had I done to him? What had I done to our life? Worst of all, what did I do to our children?

So the second day of our visit to the cancer hospital, as we were getting ready to leave the hotel room to go back to the hospital for my afternoon appointments, all I could offer both of us was to tell Dan that I should to go by myself. To sell my idea that would allow him to rest from my nightmare and allow me to rest from his pain, I said, "You would only be sitting around and waiting for me anyway." We were in quicksand and knew I could not save both of us. I knew I was in far deeper than he was. I also knew the only way I could save him from his pain was to save and heal myself first.

This thought was the beginning of me coming to know my sacred voice. This thought was the beginning of understanding that there was another way to navigate my life. This was the first time I heard the female voice of God that I thought was my own. She seemed to show up and create an opening for change at the most critical times. She would guide me with her insight to do something other than what I would have done in the past. I had no idea what was going on at the time. Then I was intrigued by my new way of thinking but had no idea where it came from. I think I was so scared and overwhelmed that I had to find a way to hear wisdom from a place beyond my own mind.

This was the first time I chose to leave a fallen comrade behind, my husband, to go get help for myself. My life's philosophy to that point had always been that I was strong enough to carry everyone and everything both physically and mentally. For the first time in my life, I now understood the implications of carrying that kind of weight on my back and in my heart. I was now mortally wounded and I knew the only way I had any chance of rescuing Dan was to save myself first. To most people that would totally make sense; to me it was a foreign thought. I had read something in a magazine that talked about putting yourself first, but I thought that people who did that or took time for themselves were self-centered. I knew some women who did this and I was very judgmental of their selfish behavior. It turned out that my selfish, *less than* mind that never allowed me to take time for myself was trying to take me out for the rest of my family's lives.

When I began my cancer journey, I did not fight cancer bravely or courageously. I fought it through the all-encompassing fear of my human experience.

After my CAT scan, blood draws, medical record reviews, and examinations it was early afternoon on the third day of our trip to the cancer hospital. Dan and I were meeting with my assigned oncologist for the first time. The leading item on her agenda was showing me, on an Internet calculator, my survival odds with and without doing chemo. If I didn't do chemo, there would be a sixty percent chance of the cancer returning. If I did do chemo, there would be a thirty-five percent chance of it returning. The part of the calculation that she left out was that if I was in the seventy-five percent group that would not have their tumor completely eliminated by the chemo that my life odds were really no better than if had I not done the chemo… and maybe worse.

When fear has you adding your kids' lives without you to your mortality percentage, you lose track of the mathematical fact that at best chemo for triple-negative breast cancer works on twenty-five percent of the people who get it. You never make it to the bottom-line percentage that three out of every four people who have stage II triple-negative breast cancer the size of mine with at least one lymph node affected, will not be saved by the chemo. I was always good at mental math, but overwhelming anxiety shuts down your ability to calculate your future. I had no capacity at that moment to even count to ten, so I just nodded my head.

Later as I became increasingly sicker from the chemo, I wondered what percentage group I would be placed in if I died from the chemo.

I decided they would most likely put me in the not-coming-back percentage since it certainly would have stopped any chance of that.

After the chemo pre-sale demo, the doctor presented my options. I could choose to do either surgery or chemo first. My thought that I wanted to research chemo more before making a decision was not thrown into the corral as a choice. Apparently, all sheep with triple-negative breast cancer need chemo.

I chose surgery. I just wanted the cancer out. My tumor was out of control and growing. I knew I was out of control too and somehow thought I could regain my composure if this lump wasn't sitting inside of me for one more second. I did not want it to remind me of my failure and that I was *less than* everyone else every second of the day. I wanted to cut it out in hope that my fear and failure would be removed with it. Out of sight, out of mind. That's the way I rolled. Remove any part of me that was *less than* and move on. With my decision to remove the tumor, I was sent to speak with my assigned surgeon. I really liked him. He was an old-school doctor, one who cared and had as much time for you as you needed, one who listened first and spoke after, one who gave you the full details of his answer and then asked if you wanted to know more. I immediately felt sure I wanted him to be my surgeon.

Errrr—that damn record again. Just as we were discussing what my new, improved, cosmetically enhanced breasts would look like, the surgeon suddenly noticed something in my CAT scan report revealing an abnormality in one of my vertebrae that could indicate that the cancer had already spread to my bones. There it was again, "*Dant-dant-da!*" Within five minutes of that discovery, the oncologist, who had thoroughly covered my need for chemo yet missed the vertebrae detail, came back to discuss my now singular option. The previously open door to our examination room was shut as she entered.

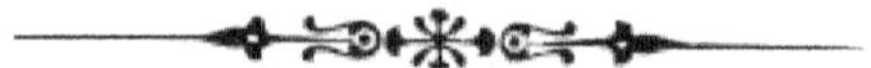

I could always make everything look like it was under control when I had my salesman's game face on. Now the business of being me was failing. With all the tears, my mascara was smearing, my eyeliner was running, and my lipstick was washed away. My game face was falling apart. I could not even think, let alone speak. Then I fell for the oldest sales trick in the book: create a need for your product by generating fear in the customer.

I was now in a B movie, where the patient is told the results are worse than expected. I vividly recalled a black-and-white television show I watched when I was a kid, remembering the words spoken by a doctor in a white coat that were delivered in a deep, finalizing tone: "Start getting your affairs in order." My faint grip that was tenuously keeping me from falling deeper into my *less than* chasm let go. As I began to free-fall, the only words that meekly came out were, "What are the odds it has spread?" The oncologist then closed her eyes as if she was entering the question into an online calculator in her brain. As she re-opened them, she semi-emphatically stated, "Thirty percent." Upon receipt of her number, I knew it was very close to the after-chemo reoccurrence percentage number that I had heard during the chemo pre-sale pitch. That number did not feel like the truth, but I didn't know if she was lying and making it sound better or worse than it really was. Fear had paralyzed my vocal cords, and I had no ability at that moment to follow up with my thought.

Dan and I did not even look at each other after she said the number, because that would make it *real*, and we were at the tipping point of *real.* My love sat in his hard seat, and I sat on the cold examining table. With the door now shut, the vacuum created in that room stifled both of us and prohibited either of us from moving toward each other. As I sat there staring down at the floor, unable to look up, the doctor continued to talk about something. Without lifting my head, my thoughts and eyes drifted toward my beloved. I could only see the bottom portion of my husband as he sat in his chair. I was sad that I could not be next to him; I desperately wanted to hold his hand. It was then I saw that Dan, like me, had his hands entwined and clenched to each other. I looked back at my own clasped, pale hands and bulging knuckles left white from my own grip. I felt a comfort remembering that from the time I met Dan twelve years earlier we had always held on to each other and I knew that at this moment, we were holding on to each other tighter than ever before.

The doctor eventually left the room. I rose from the table to get my things together, making small talk with Dan but avoiding all direct eye contact. I could not let him see the wildfire of fear that was now inside my bones. I had only been at this place that assured me they knew better than anyone how to cure my cancer for thirty-six hours and I had already fallen so far into my *less than* chasm that the daylight above disappeared. I wasn't yet in a wheelchair, but I was already looking down.

I was scheduled for a bone scan late that afternoon and was hooked up for my first chemo that night, before they would even have the bone-scan results back. That moment of that day, the die was cast: the moment we allowed the doctor to convince us to do chemo first. The day when fear, not fact, was the basis of our plan to move forward. We had made a life-altering decision to keep my tumor, my fear, and my failure uncomfortably screaming from inside of me.

The first step to your destination is choosing to look Over There. Fear had me too afraid to even flinch. Eventually, my world would turn allowing me to let go of my fear and finally stop being enclosed by the machine of cancer.

The life or death confirmation machine was located in the underground portion of the hospital, so it did not matter that the window I looked out, as I descended the stairs heading to my bone scan test, provided a view of the impending evening darkness. Yet, I still noted the nightfall anyway. I had never been in any machine in my life before the apparatus I had disappeared into twenty-four hours prior. That machine had produced an image of a shadowed vertebrae in my back that cast a deeper shade of darkness over my yawning chasm. Now I had to enter another, similar, machine that was going to again surround and cover three-quarters of the length of my body, limiting my intake of fresh air. I almost had a panic attack just thinking about getting in there. These machines were much more confining than that small office where I first received the big news about cancer. I decided the worse the big news gets, the smaller the space they put you into receive it.

I asked several times if there was enough air in the machine to breathe since I hadn't been able to catch my breath since my diagnosis, and now that I was inside of this hospital, I was finding even less air to try and do so. My mind was racing a thousand miles an hour and I was told that I could not so much as flinch for the next twenty minutes. I was also expected to hold my breath at different intervals throughout the test as I was not flinching. It was then I began to realize that I could not do this. It was too much; it was far more than my life skill set encompassed. The only thing that I could do for now was close my eyes, hold in my tears, take some anti-anxiety medication, and try to figure out how I was going to find my way out of the cancer machine and my nightmare.

When you are free-falling and being thrashed about, sometimes spinning, sometimes tumbling down through the darkness of the void, you no longer have your bearings to know which way up is. *How will I ever find my way out of here when I cannot think or even see which way is up?* It would not happen until I could learn how to stop flinching from my mind's attacks and could find a way to enough air into my heart and breathe. Not to know which way was up but to find the stillness I needed to find God, who was my only way out.

I felt like I was a contestant in The Hunger Games, hoping medicine would drop from the sky while wandering through an ever-changing labyrinth. I was constantly stumbling into corners where death lurked, waiting to grab me. I was in so much fear that I desperately kept trying to find my way back from where I came, thinking that somehow something had changed Here. It never occurred to me that if I could just remember what I forgot, the way out would be would be found Over There.

Three weeks after hearing the big news in that small office, my world shrank even more, moving me closer to the light switch. The only thing that had grown in those past weeks other than my fear was my tumor. So I doubled down. I began to put poison in my body, trying to kill the fear as much as the cancer. I was attempting to fix my insides with everything from the outside. My body wanted the cancer out, and my heart was working overtime in response. My mind would stop it from happening.

I do not remember much of my first chemo; it was only a matter of hours between my first meeting with the oncologist and my first injection of her best advice: chemo. I had to get a PICC line placed in my arm to allow the chemo access to my veins. I remember that was painful. Then I rode through the rest of the chemo prep assembly line of appointments. All that was required at each stop was to show my all-day Blue Cross and Blue Shield ride pass circling my wrist. Then suddenly it was 7:00 o'clock at night and I was in a room with my

PICC line hooked up to large bags of magic, being told that I was fortunate to get a last-minute spot for my first chemo.

My husband sat in a chair watching television as the bags of tumor toxins were started and finished, and then more bags of enchantment were brought in and methodically added until the last drop drained from them five hours later. I sat on a shaky bed in so much shock that this was happening to me that I could not even verbalize my horror while watching the show. As I felt the heat of the chemo permeating my entire body, I simultaneously listened to my mind mocking me for selling myself out. My numb body became stiff. I tried to pretend it wasn't happening and still thought there was a chance I might wake up from my heroic-coma nightmare. When it was over, Dan turned off the television. We now had to watch what we had done without any commercial breaks.

On the way back to the hotel, the deafening silence between Dan and me made it very clear that there was usually no singing or happy talk when you returned from the show, only on the way to the hospital. We arrived back at the hotel as weary cancer travelers and fallen rock stars. I was in stifling numbness and disbelief about what I had just done to myself, and Dan was sullen. When you are in oppressive shock and your husband is immersed in despair, the omnipresent weight leaves you both lying on a hotel room bed unable to speak. When you both think that one of you is going to die, knowing that part of both of you already has, you breathe in sorrow and exhale loneliness. We both felt like we had participated in something unspeakably wrong trying to hold on to what we had. Desperately begging someone to let us stay together while at the same time silently mouthing the word *goodbye*. We left the cancer hospital like washed-up rock star junkies caught with drugs abroad, returning home in handcuffs.

PART 3

Thrashing In The Chasm

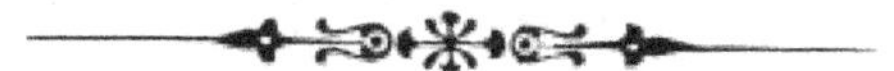

What you sometimes forget when you think you have mastered the game of winning is how easy it becomes to underestimate the strength of your opponent in the next round.

After returning from the first chemo and knowing that only the fear, but not the cancer, had spread to my bones, I kept marching further down the only trail I knew. I had a few of the chemo side effects that my cancer handbook described but was able to sleep most of them off pretty easily. My hair, still attached to my head, allowed me to look in the mirror and pretend everything could still be the same. My chemo fatigue allowed me to look in the mirror and imagine that numbness had now replaced fear.

The tumor shrank considerably almost immediately. Yes, my mantra cards worked! The walnut-sized lump in my breast was seventy-five percent gone. I thought I was doing what I always did: winning. I was doing what I did best—overcoming adversity and taking control. I was starting to believe in the magic of chemotherapy and two weeks later went back for round two. This time my hotel room was closer to the hospital and I only took my small suitcase.

The day prior to my second chemo, I had a port device surgically placed in my upper left chest above my heart so I would no longer need a PICC line in my arm to receive chemo. They told me to do this because it is less painful than getting a PICC line in your arm every time you have chemo. They said I should do this because it reduces the chances of getting blood clots that could cost me my life. Being a sheep with good insurance, I agreed.

I received the deluxe model port with dual discs so I could have two needles inserted into me at the same time, allowing me to take in two bags of liquid magic simultaneously. The port device's dual-discs were surgically implanted beneath my left collar bone. The two-inch scar and now empty space that was carved out for it remains today. It is not a badge of courage; it is simply another reminder of my ruthless war.

The port's catheter tube was threaded into one of the large veins in my neck and descended through my chest stopping near the top of my heart. Every time I turned my head, the vein in my neck would try to bend with my movement but the plastic tube inside of it could not. So they were right; I no longer had pain on the day they placed the PICC line in my arm for chemo. I now felt like I was being strangled every time I tried to turn my head. I was now branded not just by the scar but also by the device itself protruding out from my chest for the entire world to see that cancer looked as painful as it felt.

The one thing that my intuition was right about was that cancer wasn't my thing. It became apparent very quickly after my second chemo that cancer really was not my thing. I was terrible at having cancer! You always read in the obituaries about how people "courageously fought" their cancers—how they "bravely battled" cancer. My obituary would have read, "She was an inept fighter whose constant blows to herself fanned the flames of the fire burning beneath her. Cancer really was not her thing. Too bad she didn't have a heart attack; at least she would not have caught on fire."

Desperation and fear are swirling around you as you continue digesting toxins that are eliminating your red and white blood cells along with your tumor cells. The nurses who give it to you are suited up from head to toe with thick plastic masks and rubber gloves. They are afraid of getting even a single drop of the very chemicals they are pumping directly into your body on themselves.

Once the chemo fills your body, it circulates through your heart, brain, and every vital organ, carried by your own blood over and over. Your immune system is wiped out, leaving you vulnerable to the slightest of germs. Your entire body is stripped of all of your hair, including your eyebrows, eyelashes, arms, and nose hair, leaving you more naked than a baby. Your esophagus and stomach lining cells are eaten away by the chemo, leaving you with nausea. The residue of the chemo makes your saliva taste as if you are sucking on dirty pennies and nickels. You desperately try to get that filthy taste out of your mouth. You put anything you can in your mouth to try to get rid of the nasty taste for just one second. That is until you get ulcers in your mouth, and then you will not put anything in your mouth, including food.

Your stools turn hard as rocks and cut your rectum on the way out. That is if you can get it out, until a couple of days later when you will not be able to keep any of it in. The bones in your feet lock up and cramp as you try to walk; then your toenails fall off, leaving open wounds. Your hips ache so bad, making you feel like they might snap at any moment. The nerves in your eyes and your extremities become damaged and numb leaving you unable to tell where you begin or end. The chemo confuses your thinking, and you are not even sure you are still really here. The steroids that you take right before and after receiving chemo to counteract its side effects have their own side effect of causing your face to swell up like a balloon and turn yellow. They also have another effect: making you angry. You then become more enraged with yourself for putting this poison in your body than for getting cancer in the first place. But the worst part of the steroid support is that it stops you from sleeping through the chemo nightmare for three days. You then sit up all night by yourself and cry. The chemo cocktail actually makes you to cry… more than you ever have in your life. The stench of chemo turns your stomach as it slows your mind. All of this leaves you only thinking one thing about yourself: you are a cancer sheep.

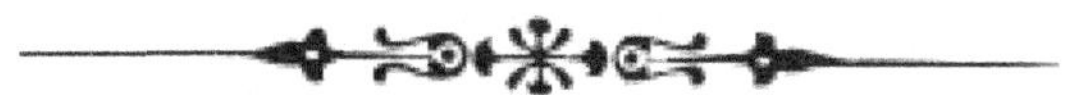

What is Truth? Truth is what you know without consideration. Truth resides in simplicity. It just is. Truth sits comfortably and is at peace within you. There is a lot of space and air around Truth. Truth is known from the place of your holiness. There are a lot of things that are true. The sun comes up in the morning. This is true, but the majesty in the rising of the sun is Truth. Anytime you are given a peek of your perfection in something you hear, see, or feel; Truth is there. That is why when a child smiles at you, Truth is stirred in you. It reminds you of who you really are… a part of God.

After returning from my second chemo, the illusion in the mirror changed. As I looked in the mirror and ran my hands through my full blonde hair, it became entangled within my fingers and fell to the floor. Handful after handful of my prideful hair left me with the exact same motion that I had used to run my hands through it thousands of times before. This time the relationship had changed. My hair could no longer be separated by my fingers and could not hold on even with the gentlest of my human touch. Today, as I looked in the mirror, I could see that everything about what I thought I saw before was falling away and would never be the same. Now, looking into the mirror, the numbness that had been masking my fear had been shaken awake by the intensity of my all-encompassing mental and physical pain.

After my second chemo and port insertion, my body was wrung out. There turned out to be a juggling act at the magic show. It was called "Let's have your body find enough white and red blood cells to recover from the chemo we put into you, try to heal around this device we sewed into you, and then try to find a way to eliminate tumor cells from your body simultaneously." I was wiped out and could not stand up for more than a few seconds without becoming so nauseous from my fatigue that I would almost pass out. Whenever I could force myself to eat, within five minutes every bit of it would shoot out of my butt at lightning speed and bring significant amounts of blood with it. I could not walk. Every step felt like I no longer had padding on the bottom of my feet and my bones were directly rubbing against the floor. Red stuff was coming out of my ears, and my nose would bleed most of the day. I was not doing well and I knew it. When I went back to Chicago for my third chemo treatment, I told them I needed to take a break from the chemo.

Prior to going to the cancer hospital in Chicago, a surgeon in Fargo had told me that having surgery after two rounds of chemo was one of my options. I, however, wanted to be operated on by the old-school surgeon in Chicago. My assigned oncologist in Chicago whom I needed approval from for the surgery spent thirty minutes telling me to do otherwise. I had even brought my mother to my appointment so she could stick up for me and tell the doctor to stop the chemo. I asked and was told that the effectiveness of the chemo would not be changed by doing surgery now, but I was still told to stay the course. I promised over and over I would finish the chemo after surgery but the oncologist did not believe me. Every issue and reason I gave for being physically unable to do another chemo was poo-pooed away by the doctor. I was treated like a whiney recruit at basic training who needed to toughen up and complete the obstacle course. The doctor was an impenetrable force and would not yield to my request. I was too weak and did not win this round in the fight for my life.

Months later, after suffering the extreme consequences of losing that battle, I was told by that physician in Chicago that she did not grant my request, because the chemo had been so successful. After my second chemo, the tumor could no longer be felt. Everyone was so amazed at my success. I wanted to walk away from the roulette wheel with my winnings, knowing I was not physically able to do a third chemo. I wanted to do surgery and clear any remains of the cancer. The doctor wanted to double down and spin the wheel again. I was just a sheep and she was the house, so her rules trumped mine and my appeal was denied. It was my right to have surgery, and that oncologist took it from me because I had no brain cells, no physical ability, and no Truth to stand with. She was afraid I would not do more chemo if I had done the surgery then. Well, she got her way; I ended up doing much, much more chemo because I did not have the surgery I begged for. I did the third chemo. Letting her truth reign over mine in that room that day almost killed me.

The Truth does not cease to be because you do not choose to embrace it. The Truth that I should not have had that third chemo did not change because I chose to surrender to what was untrue. I gave up on my Truth and allowed myself to suffer greatly through that doctor's white-coated truth. At that time, I did not understand what it meant to know Truth and how to sit in it without compromise, and it almost cost me my life. Not holding on to your Truth can create small ripples in your life or create a wave that concedes your life. When you get to the point where you let go of your Truth one too many times like I did, you have hit the climax of your story.

I had a front-row seat to watch what my family's life would be like without me. I clearly witnessed the unrelenting pain that broke my sons' little hearts, caused by losing the only mother they had ever known. How does a kid go to school and through his day when his mom, his strong mom who does everything, can't even get off the couch and cries all the time? When Grandma comes and stays and stays? I was always trying so hard to protect my sons from everything, while doing anything for them, that I forgot to protect the thing they needed the most: me. I continuously punished myself as I sat in my less than chasm, thinking that my big miscalculation would cause one of the most hurtful and saddest things that could ever happen to a kid: having your mom die.

Every morning my mom would get the kids up and ready for school. As I heard everyone's day starting, I would tell myself to get downstairs so the kids could see me before they went to school, hoping that they would believe I was okay. I would put on my blonde hair halo piece, my red baseball cap on top of it, get my pain in check, summon up any and all energy I could find, and begin my slow walk down the stairs, holding on to the handrail for dear life. I would tell myself that I needed to sit on the couch upright for fifteen minutes or so before they left for school and act as if I was fine, thinking that if I could just sit up they would overlook all the otherwise horrifying parts of my condition and go to school thinking I was okay. Most days I could put on the charade; some days I would just lie there… a couple of days I could not even get out of bed.

From the couch, I would watch the three of them at the breakfast table, seeing and hearing their pain as all of their hearts were breaking. I would try not to think about the fact that my kids knew that I could not even stand, let alone get the cereal, bowls, spoons, and milk out for them anymore.

I would watch my mom's heroic effort to make up for everything that I was not doing for my children by doing everything she could to have a smooth morning. Yet every day I would hear my youngest son Sam get angry with her. He would talk back and be obstinate as she asked him to do all the things he used to do for me.

Sam would continue to get more frustrated and more defiant with each request from my mom. I knew that all he needed in order to calm down was for his mom, not my mom, to pour milk into his cereal bowl for him. My older son Daniel tried to hide the uneasiness in our house by becoming even more agreeable than usual. He also started demanding that type of obedience from Sam. They would often get into yelling and physical fights because Daniel wanted Sam to behave better. Daniel was upset because when his mom couldn't pour milk into his cereal bowl for him, he thought everyone needed to hold their sadness in and act better to help her get better.

My mom did not want me to worry about them. She wanted me to think that what was happening to me was not affecting them. She wanted me to think that what was happening to me was not affecting her.

I knew my boys were both reacting to something they could not understand. How could they when I could not grasp it either. The sadness, anger, and confusion spewing from my kids' loss of their safety and security, which I could no longer provide, created a heavy, negative, foreboding energy in our house, causing me to sink even deeper into my *less than* chasm.

Before cancer, my sons and I would always be joking and laughing as we were running out the door to take them to school in the morning. Now when they left, it was a quiet march away from me, knowing that I would not be picking them up from school either, not even knowing if I would be there or at the hospital when they returned home.

Now when the door closed behind them each morning, unable to stand the constriction of the lie for one more second, I would whip off my hat and fake hair halo within seconds and immediately fall onto the couch from exhaustion. I would make sure my propaganda was back in place on my head at 3:00 o'clock when school was over so I could resume my charade. Over and over I would beg myself to sit up for fifteen minutes after they arrived so they could think that I had been fine all day and feel free to go off to play with their friends.

Everyone in our house was lost and fumbling within the dark cloud of cancer. I was in the full throws of terror and living the horror the nightmare brought. My husband was in stone-cold denial. I watched him become robotic. Dan would get up early, go to work, go to the grocery store, make dinner, clean the house, make small talk with my mom, do the kids' homework, and then sit in his chair next to his wife with her cheek stuck to the fake leather couch. He could not bear to discuss anything about my sickness. Dan was too close to the edge of losing me, and talking about it would push him over. I watched him wander through the dark days, mostly in shock and disassociation with my cancer, going through the motions, to keep our family churning.

She gave me life and was the one person who spent the most time with me during cancer helping me save my life. My mom has always been and will always be the wind beneath my wings.

Something old, something new, something borrowed, something blue. Something old represents continuity. It comes first because it represents where your roots have been planted. My past held the stores of the nourishing love that I needed. My family and friends who were a part of my history brought the remembrance of the riches of the love from my yesterdays to me now. Those who had years of abundant time with me brought me the deep-seated, longstanding love that supported me through the winds of my storm. They reminded me of my innocence as well as my growth. They brought me love through laughter at my past follies and theirs. They reminded me of the sacred times of my Truth that I had forgotten.

My mom is my most important *something old.* My fondest memories of her include: sewing clothes for my Barbies, driving me to deliver my paper route every Sunday because the papers were always heavy, making homemade pizza before my high school basketball games, typing my college papers while trying to decipher my messy handwriting, *and* being my most constant and secure lifeline during cancer.

During my illness, after my mom returned from taking the kids to school, the house became quiet. I spent most of my time on the living room couch. At first trying to figure out how to cure my cancer and live a long life, but eventually mostly crying and trying to figure out how to find a way to make it through the rest of the day. My mom wasn't sure how much of herself to inject, never knowing what I would need on any given day. She would wash the morning dishes, do a few loads of laundry, and come in and out of the living room, wanting to give me my space and at the same time be there for me.

I knew Mom felt confined in our house that was now half its original size since we were right in the middle of remodeling it when I got sick. Knowing our construction meant she had to sleep on a couch in our old tattered family room weighed on me. Knowing that the kids were behaving badly made me feel worse. I felt guilty and would often apologize to my mom for taking her away from the calm of her well-deserved retirement to pick up the mess I had made of my life. I felt my being sick was a terrible burden to put on her. I was supposed to be there for her, not the other way around.

She never complained though. She repeatedly listened and listened and listened to me throughout my search for answers—from what the Internet said, what someone told me, what books I ordered but was now too sick to read, what pills I needed to take and what supplements would ease their side effects, to what hurt now, where and how it hurt, what I was going to try to force myself to eat, when my next appointment was, my anger at the doctors, disdain for myself, frustration with my kids' behavior, and on and on.

I got sick of hearing myself, but she patiently and lovingly listened to everything I kept spewing over and over and over. How was I going to get myself out of this mess? Every failed thought or plan she usually heard twice. She would always sit next to me, holding my hand and listening to me as I continued to spiral deeper and deeper into the abyss. Then, when I could not find any words, she would allow me to cry and cry because many days that is all I could do. She sat with me in my desperation, not showing hers, day after day, week after week, month after month.

I never needed to ask her for comfort because her love was always warmly wrapped around me like a soft and familiar sweater. She was present and available for me no matter what, helping me navigate whatever was happening at that moment. When I didn't know how to make me better, her love would always make me *feel* better.

I know a lot of the times I would not be making any sense or would be so lost in my sadness and isolation that both of us were incapable of understanding what was going on. She knew in those moments that there were no answers to be found. She also knew that the most important thing in those moments was not looking for a way out for me, but being there to listen and care about what I was experiencing. She sat right next to me as I lay in my unknown and scary depths. I learned that, while you are waiting for an answer, sometimes you just need someone to hold the moment open for you to breathe. Mom did that for me. Without my mom, I would not have had the ability to exhale through my storm. She helped me find calmness in my tempest by allowing me to unload the chaos from my mind. She was my home base and my most crucial and solid lifeline that held on to me as I thrashed about in my chasm.

Along with my family, my friend Judy is also one of my dearest *something olds*. She was not only my first friend when I moved to California, but at the end of my thirteen-year stay there, she was still one my best friends. She says we are soulmates. I agree.

I met her when I applied for a position at a software company. She hired me and then almost immediately adopted me as her younger sister. Judy has been a significant part of my life for over seventeen years and has always been someone on whom I could count to catch me when I was falling. Her importance only grew during cancer. She would check in on me but more importantly she would answer her phone when I called… always. She used her words to put one arm around my shoulder and with her compassion she held my shaking hand.

The times when I was able to work on putting the pieces of my puzzle together; Judy would roll up her sleeves, always ready to help. When you've known someone so long, sometimes they know you, in some ways, better than you know yourself. They can recognize things about you through their love for you that you are missing. They can help you find that puzzle piece you've been looking for but searching too intently to find. Judy, in her patient, teaching way, was able to help me see things I couldn't understand as well as talk through things that I thought I did, so that I could change my mind. She was my guiding spiritual hand and life coach when my game was in real trouble. She lovingly steered me in whatever direction I needed to go, helping me pick up my wrecked self. Judy knew that the only person who could get me out of my *less than* chasm was me. She also knew that a good friend could point you in the right direction.

PART 4

Choosing Life

For the most part, I was too sick to watch television. I mostly stared into the nothingness of my surroundings. For some reason, the television was on in my hospital room without the volume, and footage of a building being demolished caught my eye. This was not the first time I had seen a building implode on the news, but my intrigue with the sight of the total destruction was still the same. I remembered seeing a news clip from years before when it was explained how experts strategically placed explosives throughout a fated structure. The devices were then set off in a planned sequence so the building would break down in fundamentally important locations first. This was done knowing that the essential failures would cascade forward until their accumulated weight hit a critical mass, causing the simultaneous collapse of the remaining structure. Everything from the first explosion through the last shred of dust ended up in a pile of ash on the ground with a cloud of smoke hanging in the air, covering the remains from sight. The resulting nothingness had once been something that was majestically conceived, rendered with a vision, precisely designed, calculated as worthy, built with strength and ingenuity, and judged to be safe. The construction's purpose was intended to let life enter and abide. Then it was no more… reduced to ashes in a matter of seconds; a once great composition leveled on an ordinary sunny morning.

I woke up again sick, sick, sick. This was the third time I had had chemo, and I thought I knew how it worked. Day three through day six face-planted in the couch, yes—but not day eight being worse than ever. Having learned some of the tricks of the chemo trade to curb the multitude of physical issues that arose, I couldn't believe I was going down so hard for so long. I was well-armed with steroids, anti-nausea meds, Senokot, Clariton, every supplement under the sun, emu oil, petroleum jelly, and mouthwash. I cannot remember everything, but I was doing it all.

I was at home alone since my mom had had to leave for a week. I thought I would be able to take care of myself while she was gone. I remember getting up that morning and telling myself that I just was not trying hard enough. I was going to do better and do everything perfectly that day. *Maybe if I got everything exactly right, I would feel better. If I could just eat something, if I could just sit up, if I could just take all my supplements today, if I could just be better at doing this; maybe I would not be so sick. I am a good sheep following the cancer rules and trying so hard to do everything right, so why am I so sick?*

Two hours after that discussion with myself, I had to ask, "Why do I now have a fever?" I had been warned about this in the cancer rulebook. Rule Number 1: you cannot have a fever, since chemo kills your white blood cells leaving your body unable to fight any type of infection. *Okay, let's find a thermometer.* This takes time when you can't walk upright and can't remember where *you* are, let alone where the thermometer is. Fifteen minutes later; *Okay 103.5. Not good. Rule*

Number 2: if your temperature is above 100.5, you must immediately go to the emergency room. I lay there realizing that I could no longer do enough things right to make myself better and reluctantly I called my husband home from work.

I had always been really good at getting my way; making a plan and winning. This was the beginning of a big losing streak for the golden girl. I had no idea where I was headed, and if I had, I would have passed and taken the next train out of cancer city. Instead, I dislodged from the ledge in my *less than* chasm and fell down deeper.

At the emergency room in Jamestown, not only did I have a really high temperature, I had a really weak pulse. When I rolled over in the hospital bed as the physician was examining me, my husband noticed that most of my left butt cheek was red and told the doctor. The medical practitioner looked closer. He found a raging infection. The doctor then said I was too sick for my husband to drive me the ninety miles to a better hospital in Fargo where they could cut the infection out of my body. By the time the ambulance got me to the hospital in Fargo, my blood pressure had dropped even further. As they began prepping me for surgery, an older nurse said, "If you had waited until tomorrow to come in, you would definitely not have made it." I didn't have the strength or the courage to ask her what that meant in terms of me coming in today.

Then someone mistakenly let my kids in the room. When I saw the shock and terror on their little faces as they gazed at me, I knew that I had been hurt while trying to perform a heroic act. Not by attempting to save anyone else, just myself. Their tear-filled, scared, and lonely faces looked as I imagined they would if they were at my funeral and staring at me in the casket. I started to cry because I could not bear to see those expressions of pain on my children's faces. They were then scurried out of the room and I was taken to surgery.

Once in the operating room, I heard the medical team talking about having two patients coming in for emergency surgery and one's blood pressure was very low. I thought, *Hello, that's me. Does that mean I'm going to die?* Once again, I did not really want to know the answer. After surgery, I was told that I had Methicillin-resistant Staphylococcus aureus (MRSA), a dangerous staph infection. I was also told that I had very few white blood cells, which were necessary for my immune system to stop it. No amount of antibiotics will thwart an infection, let alone one of the worst infections, without white blood cells. I thought, *Seriously, is there any good news in this place?* It's a good thing I was too incoherent to grasp the severity of the situation and quickly fell back into my delirium.

At one point during my first night in the hospital, when things were dicey at best, I woke up startled, sensing someone standing next to my bed. I was lying flat on my back and turned my head to the right see who was beside me. *Ahhh, it's my dead father.* He was way too visible to me at that moment and his presence scared me. I thought he was there because I was dying. In my delirium I said, "Dad, you're more than welcome to stand there, but I'm not going anywhere with you!"

I then turned my head back to face forward with tears forming in my eyes, and asked God to let me make it through the night. I murmured, "Please let me live." I think I passed out after that.

The worst was yet to come. It wasn't the surgery, the deep open hole left by the removal of the MRSA abscess, the MRSA still in my body, the mega doses of antibiotics, high fever, relentless nausea, or all the other chemo-related physical issues that took me to my breaking point. It was diarrhea. As embarrassing as it sounds, the big D was what made everything too much to take. I had diarrhea as often as every fifteen minutes for three days and nights. My bowels were releasing excrement all over me again and again. Although I now understand that my mind had been metaphorically doing this to me every day prior to this, the actual physical expression of it was too much. I may have been able to hold back my mind's offensive subconscious stuff with my *more than* shield, but my *less thans* had now seeped out into conscious foul stuff that I was unable to stop with anything.

As diarrhea occurred again and again, it became too much. I had to trade in the last of my dignity as I over and over had to tell the nurses it happened again. Once more having to ask for help to take off my gown, now full of my *less than* personal mess, and ask for assistance to walk the four feet to the bathroom, too dizzy to do so on my own. Once in the bathroom, unable to stand, I would crouch over in the shower as I tried to hose myself off with the hand held shower head. I cried under my breath from the stinging of the spraying water as it ran over the open hole in my butt that had MRSA in it, and now every gross thing you can imagine from my intestines in it too. I sobbed out loud from the pain in my mind as it was losing more and more control in lockstep with the loss of my dignity in the world.

I had never really been seriously sick or in the hospital overnight other than having my kids. Cancer and its entourage overwhelmed my understanding of illness. From the moment of my diagnosis, the pelting horror of the mental and physical assault never stopped. The intensity that started as snow blowing around the top of the mountain was now an avalanche that swept me under and gathered speed as my descent continued. In a short seven weeks, I had not even found a way to hold my grip around my original cancer diagnosis, and now I lay in the unknown depths of my dark gorge, choking on chemo and MRSA, unable to breathe or think.

What I didn't know about cancer was deadly. As I sat in the surgical unit of the hospital, I did not even know they had a separate cancer floor of the hospital and that with my compromised immunity I should have been there. I also did not know that a surgical resident student, who expected me to get better when my body was so immune-compromised, should not have been allowed to make decisions regarding my care.

On my third day in the hospital a young surgical resident came into my room at 5:30 a.m., abruptly woke me from my sleep and told me that I needed to leave the hospital. Firmly holding her impenetrable clipboard in front of her heart, she told me that I should have been better by now. Other people with abscesses left in one or two days. Apparently this surgical intern had not done an oncology rotation. I told her I thought due to taking chemo and my lack of white blood cells it was taking me longer. Her self-justifying reply was that if that was the case I still needed to leave the hospital because of all the potential infections that I could get from being there.

In less than two months from hearing the dreadful word *cancer*, I had been rounded up with the other cancer sheep, sheared of my dignity that allowed me to run through life on my terms, and now was being dragged out of the corral by an arrogant medical student in a starchy white coat. She thought because someone was good at anatomy and physiology they knew how to heal people. In truth she was only someone whose ignorance about healing surpassed mine.

I had never been a shrinking violet and was a mighty force to challenge. My whole life I not only fought my battles but also stood up for those who could not stand up for themselves. Now, for the first time, I had to bow down out of weakness, both physical and mental, and beg this uncaring clinician through my tears to allow me to stay in the hospital for one more day. I knew how sick I was and I had to plead with her to let me stay and get more intravenous antibiotics that I felt I needed to save my life. There is nothing more merciless and demeaning to another human being than requiring them to beg you for their life. This humiliation took the last bit of what propped me up in the world and kicked it out from under me. That's when I broke. I was too sick to acknowledge it that day as I could only focus on trying not to die. Later my mind would reveal to me what this wolf in a white sheep's clothing had done by dragging me out of the corral to the slaughter.

The next day I went home loaded with oral antibiotics. I knew I should have been in the hospital, but my new career as a sheep left me unable to negotiate that type of deal. My exile on my couch only lasted for one day. The morning of my second day at home I went back to the emergency room and was again admitted to the hospital and put on intravenous antibiotics with a second MRSA abscess that needed to be surgically removed.

I later found out that the first MRSA abscess was less than a half inch from entering my rectum. The MRSA lesions were spread across most of my left butt cheek, but the one that had formed an abscess and needed to be cut out was a half inch away from becoming unstoppable if it compromised my rectum. I bowed my head as I now fully understood the meaning of the words, "Life is a game of inches and but for the grace of God go I."

Surviving required me to unconditionally seize the full depth of my experiences. This created the transformative circumstance necessary for restoration.

After my second round with MRSA, I was told that there was now a high chance that I would be a MRSA carrier for the rest of my life. In the long run, that would matter. In my present, which did not guarantee any future, it was an enormous burden added onto my day. To reduce the chance of being a carrier by fifty percent, I had to cover every inch of my body every day for five days with pink MRSA medicine. I found out this type of cleansing was a much more complex effort than I imagined. It's not like a shower where you let the water run down your body and mix in with the soap assuming that the combination will eventually hit all the places on you by the time it makes it to your feet. That approach to cleansing allows you to only put a special effort into cleaning the most obvious parts of you.

When you are using MRSA medicine, which has a consistency of a watered-downed lotion, you have to rub it on thoroughly from your head to your toes. You have to cover all the places on your body, even the ones you thought were impossible to reach. I had to find places on me that I had not seen or thought about in years. The prominent places on my body were no more important in this exercise than the ones I never paid attention to. I needed to take care to be wholly covered with that pink solution if it was going to work. Any small patch that I missed would mean MRSA could remain and grow, eventually and once again, enveloping my body.

After I scrubbed and covered every inch of my body starting at the top of my head and working my way to my toes with the medicine, I then had to stand in the tub/shower for seven minutes, letting it soak into the pores of my skin. Those last seven minutes were absolutely the worst, most onerous, unwelcome part of my day. I would uncomfortably stand there for what seemed like an eternity. I was so sick I would often have to sit down on the edge of the tub when I got too tired or too nauseated to stand. I would always say to myself as I was trying to do my seven minutes that the process would not be so bad if I weren't so sick. I kept thinking it would be a lot easier to heal myself if I just felt better.

I now smile at the irony of wanting to wait to heal yourself until you feel better, knowing that to feel better you need to heal yourself. I also know the uncomfortableness of my pain was the necessary and true catalyst for my change. It's easy to sit in the familiar pain your mind inflicts on you when you are mostly unaware of it but when the volume is turned up on that pain due to your intense physical pain it forces you to finally pay attention to it. Not just to relieve the discomfort, but to live. I can now look back and see the necessity and sacredness of feeling my pain and cleaning every piece of me. Immersing myself in my remedy, regardless of how uncomfortable it was, for as long as was required to fully heal. Even though this exercise did not heal my MRSA vulnerability, it helped me recognize that I needed to heal all the parts of myself, even my hidden parts, to cure my cancer.

I raise my hand to God and I choose life. Not from my mind, not from my heart, but from the place beneath my breath where my moment begins. In a place so sacred, so deep, and so quiet that you might not ever know it's there. I always

secretly hoped there might be a place like that inside. I found that just leaning into the possibility and believing in the place of Truth was all that was required to reveal the divine.

I was not humbled by the weakness cancer treatment wrought upon my mind and body; I was humbled when I received God's instantaneous and enveloping love and acceptance at the moment I asked. I was humbled knowing that I was part of something so endless and loving.

Two weeks after my second release from the hospital for MRSA and eight weeks since starting chemo, I did my fourth and supposed final A/C (Adriamycin and Cytoxan) chemo in Fargo the day after my forty-eighth birthday. Four days later, when I was again severely depleted of white blood cells, I started to notice MRSA lesions forming and again went to the emergency room in Fargo.

After being examined in the emergency room, where they found more MRSA, I was given a prescription for more medication. I was so weak from my latest chemo and now again from the MRSA that I could not walk to the hospital's pharmacy. I was given a wheelchair for my mom to take me to pick up the medicine. While I was waiting for it to be filled, I sat, decimated by the unending assault of chemo and MRSA upon my body. The wheels on the chair were locked and so were the wheels in my mind. The only thing spinning was my sadness and desperation. My bald head was exposed and I was doubled over, unable to hold my torso up, so sick that all I could do was meekly cry. It wasn't even three months since I had stood in the lobby of the cancer hospital in Chicago in the shoes of a woman who could not even fathom in her worst nightmare ever being the woman bent over in a wheelchair. As I sat there, I again thought that the woman in the wheelchair was going to die. While I was hunched over quietly sobbing, a hospital volunteer came over to me and asked me if she could get me something. I could not lift my head or form any words to speak but slowly moved my head left and right signaling no and continued to quietly cry. She didn't ask any more questions. She just started praying out loud for me and asked God to take care of me and my pain. That beautiful woman provided for me what no doctor had considered and what no pill contained. She offered me compassion through prayer and bestowed upon me love, the medicine of God.

Two days after that I woke up sicker than the night before. I knew I would be. I had started running a fever as evening set in and knew it would only keep getting worse. I already knew that when you do not have many white blood cells and get sick, your body cannot help you. I should have gone to the emergency room at that point but could not muster the mental wherewithal to go back to the hospital again in the darkness.

Through the night my insides were boiling out of control. In my disorientation and dreams I could not and would not let go of the life I had created *here*. I had to hold on to any shred of safety I had. I didn't realize that I had created all my insurance policies in a hazardous place. The safety I had accumulated in my education, my job, my bank account, my looks, and all of my possessions, including the most important one, my family, was all I had between me and extinction by fear. I was not going to unclench my white-knuckled hands to let go of any of it. I was crying from the pain of my mind's grip on those things more than from the items themselves. Even with my hand clenched, it was all disappearing: my hair, my face, my body, my mind, my money, my career. In the morning I was left with the realization that all I had left to hold on to was my family.

My relentless night and fever left me so drained and dizzy that I had to crawl backwards, on my hands and knees, down the stairs. At the bottom of the stairs I could only halfway stand up to take the necessary few steps before lunging for the couch. I told my husband and Mom that I now had to go back to the hospital. Now knowing exactly where the thermometer was, I quickly verified my temperature; it was 104.5.

When you are that sick, your body can not stand up. It is incapable. I leaned on my husband to get to the minivan. Once inside, I then had to crawl to the third-row bench seat to lie down. As I was on my hands and knees, struggling to move forward, which was really backward, I thought, *I'm not even sure there is anything left of me that is worth fighting for.* I wholly accepted the thought, and for the first time did not want to fight anymore. I lost hope. I was beginning to let go.

My husband began the 90-mile drive to the emergency room in Fargo. When you are that sick, you really cannot talk, move, or think. All you can do is stare. You can *view* life; you just cannot participate physically or mentally. Life is on television and all you can do is watch.

Every once in a while a thought would pass through my mind, but not too often. Just as your body's capacity to move is lost, so is your brain's.

I lay there curled up in the back seat of our minivan with a fever; staring, staring, staring. When thoughts shut down, all that is left is staring. All I could do was stare at my poor husband driving me to the hospital, not knowing what was next. Even though he was sitting only four feet away, my inability to speak to Dan made him seem unreachable. The man I had loved for the past twelve years had now slipped out of my weakening grip. He was now inaccessible to me. After a long while of only staring, a thought came through: *I am so sad, so alone.* I knew there wasn't much of my *less than* chasm left. Well, there was probably plenty of dark depth left, just not enough of me to remain alive for the rest of the freefall. I knew I was out of rope and the lifeline I had was now around my neck.

After another long period of staring, I somehow knew I was dying. I was so far away from the life I had known, so deep in the abyss of nothingness, that I was about to die all alone. I had never felt emptier or lonelier in all my life. I remember thinking that I never considered that dying would happen this soon or this way. I was now too lost in the nowhereness to care that I was leaving this life. I never knew what I would think as I was dying, but I didn't think as the moment was upon me that I would be too lost in the grip of my isolation to even care. I was not really fighting anything at that point. I did not even consider that it was possible for something to save me.

Everything became so distant, which felt sad on some level, but I was much more aware of the aloneness I was feeling as it was happening. I could not even find a way, as I had done from the beginning of my diagnosis, to hold on for my children's sakes. I thought about them but felt my grip on them releasing. I could simply no longer embrace them. I was too lost in the void to be with my beloved babies. They were taken from me because I had nothing left to hold on to them with. Face down in the minivan on the way to the hospital, after I'd lost my husband and my kids were then taken, I somehow decided to let go. I somehow understood that the only thing now to do was voluntarily open my hand and let the only thing I had remaining… myself… go. Simultaneously as I was letting go I thought about God. I do not know where the thought came from, and I do not think I was even a hundred percent conscious at the time. A simple thought about God was all I could form as I was incapable of asking or even hoping for anything. I was not in fear or peace. I was in the limbo of the chasm between *Here* and *Over There.* All I knew was that I was nowhere and very much alone. I did not think about what had happened or what was going to happen next. I only existed, paused in that very moment, and thought about God. It was the choice that marked the changing of the guard for who I was. Looking back, I realize that I had to find greater strength to let go than I ever did to hold on.

After the thought passed, I began to fall back into the nothingness, prepared to remain trapped within my sick body while I waited to die. But in an instant my world changed. God knew I was desperately isolated and lost inside my pain. He knew I couldn't bear my mind's suffocating aloneness as I lay there knowing that I was going to die. He knew my body was following my mind, but he heard my heart and stopped it from happening. With that simple choice: with my naked, heartfelt, honest, and unconditional choice to be with God at that moment… He came.

I began to feel comforted; a feeling of physical warmth from someone loving me. I felt a tender, soothing blanket of love on me. Through my isolation, fever, and pain, I felt a warmth radiating from a most beautiful love, making me feel cherished and worthy. There was no judgment, just a gentle, all-encompassing love, filled with overwhelming joy that I chose to be with Him.

I could not believe it. I could barely move, let alone think or talk; separating me from the world. Yet God had entered into my sealed-off space and was understanding my pain with overwhelming compassion, embracing, protecting, and taking care of me. Without judgment and with quiet peacefulness, he somehow put His words in my mind: "It's okay. I'm here for you, with you." I did not know how His voice entered my secluded world, but I knew it was real. I knew it was God.

God could have let me die alone, but His grace and love lifted me up and placed me in the palm of His hand, offering me overflowing love, tenderness, and encouragement as only a father could offer His child. He came and stopped my soul from leaving my body. I did not learn until later that preachers call this the Grace of God. God put His Grace in my mind, heart, soul, and body that day. He came to me in my greatest hour of need and hopelessness… Me, a nobody non-believer/believer. A *less than* sinner who never went to church and who had only just started praying to—or, more truthfully, begging—Him to let me live to raise my kids. He came without judgment; an abundance of mercy, love, and a humble gratefulness that I was again with Him.

I still cry when I think of how generously God showed His love for me. I did not feel worthy of even His crumbs of love, yet He offered me everything. I, who had turned away from Him for so long, could not believe how overjoyed He was to be with me. I could not believe the complete acceptance that was given with zero judgment. I had never felt such a tender and perfect love. It was far beyond the vast love I have for my own children. That kind of complete and infallible love is only known by those who again join with God and experience their Truth. I reunited with God that day and now I know the true miracle and meaning of love and life.

Once I met God and knew I was deeply loved and cherished, it was a turning point where my mind's false beliefs lost a big part of their control over me. I was no longer exclusively living in my old beliefs and chaos. Once I found God, my mind no longer had the upper hand to always make me believe I was *less than* and God was not there. After feeling loved and worthy in the eyes of God, something my unconscious beliefs never gave me, I knew God was real.

At the time, I didn't understand that my mind and the chemo had pushed me so far down into my *less than* chasm that I was leaving life *Here*, allowing me for the first time to escape it's thoughts and open up to *Over There.* Once I was with God I was able to step outside of my mind's isolation and fear: my subconscious fear of not being good enough that lay hidden beneath my successful life. The fear that required me to hold a death grip on everything, compelling me to build my web of safety and sit in its accompanying anxiety. Fear that caused me to craft my *more than* shield and hold on to it with a death grip to create a false security about life. When I was in the nothingness, about to die, I somehow found a way to let go of all of my mind's false creations so I could be with God. *"If you cling to your life you will lose it, and if you let your life go, you will save it." Luke 17:13*

As I drew closer to God, I realized that my enemy wasn't new pain; it was the fear of old pain. When your mind's fearful feelings of past hurt take over your heart, squeezing the life out of you, it's time to let them go.

"There is no fear in love; but perfect love casteth out fear." John 4:18

God saved my life in the minivan, but I still had a long way to go to heal. Since I had released my grip on everything else, God gave me something greater to embrace… His love. I had to cling to His miraculous love, because my first choice for life was just the beginning of finding all that I needed to live.

After escaping my mind *Here* and meeting God, I somehow found my way *Over There* several hours later when I again needed God. My deluxe port that was intended to allow painless access to my body for the chemo was also designed to allow easy access for any other intravenous drug or for drawing blood from my body. Despite the sales pitch working, the actual device often malfunctioned. Starting in the emergency room and continuing until five hours later in my hospital room, four nurses and one doctor all tried to draw blood from my port. This required using large needles to push great amounts of saline through it, attempting to unplug it. They then decided to try to insert an IV line as an alternative way to access my body while still trying to unplug my port. Unfortunately, since the chemo had destroyed many of my veins, they had to penetrate multiple different veins trying to find an entry into my body, piercing me over and over. After the port/IV assault had gone on for so many hours, it became too much. I could not bear the pain for one more second. I somehow left my body and went somewhere else. I exited stage right, just as I had heard people talk about on television, describing how they escaped their bodies *Here* when bad things were happening to them. Well, I took off after them and watched myself do it. The place you go to is silent. Nothing is really going on *Over There*—which I guess is the point. You are there so you do not have to be *Here.* It wasn't boring there. It was just *there.* Trust me; after staring and staring and staring, I knew monotony. Boredom is when you are in the chasm, longing to be *Here.* However, when you are *Over There,* wanting and needing to be there, it becomes somewhere safe and timeless, and not monotonous. I was beginning to appreciate having somewhere else to be besides my *less than* chasm and *Here.* I was beginning to learn how to find God.

Being *Over There* with God made me feel safe. I found that I no longer needed to react out of panic. When I felt the full safety of my being in God, my anxiety was released. It wasn't like a balloon popping; it happened peacefully, at a steady yet relaxed pace. Breath after breath, my fear dissipated. It took me a second to realize its absence and then start to embrace my calmness. I could again take long, deep, and relaxing breaths without gulping down the air through the stiffness of my frame. The spinning of my mind ceased. I received the soft power to be at ease. I was able to stop, clear, and reset my mind and body and experience peace. I was safe, wholly secure in the impenetrable circle of God. At that moment, I was not afraid. I escaped my distress. I didn't know it then—it was still to be found: the realization that fear cannot exist in the place of God.

Now I know that my stress and fear were probably more life-threatening to me than my cancer itself. When your body is stressed and fearful, the anxiety shuts down its ability to heal. That's why the day-in, day-out stress and fear of being *less than* that your mind puts on your body opens you up to illness. When you then add the worry of being sick creating more apprehension, now of dying, the cocktail becomes deadly. There are real chemical changes to how your body operates when you are under duress. The worst one is shutting down your body's repair mechanism, your immune system. When you are nervous or afraid, your body thinks it needs to focus all of its energy on giving you the strength to fight or run away from what may harm you. So your body diverts its resources from your immune system, shutting down your healing mechanisms, to give you the best chance of fighting or running away from what is threatening to harm you. Your body does not understand that your anxiety is coming from your thoughts. It thinks it is from something real, like a tiger chasing you or an avalanche coming toward you.

Tigers and avalanches are supposed to be short-term problems. Once you are safe again and you are no longer nervous or afraid, the mechanism that turned off your immune system then turns it back on for both your routine maintenance and for healing any wounds you may have received. That's why the long-term burden caused by your mind's thoughts, in addition to the constant worry created in most people's minds after the word *cancer* is pronounced on them, keeps them from healing. I had to find my way out of my mind's stress and fear, not just of being *less than* but also, now, of dying from cancer—if I was going to have any chance of healing.

Today I know that every minute my mind's stressful and fearful thoughts had me lift my heavy *more than* shield to not be *less than*, or I was afraid of dying from cancer, it was one less minute that my body was healing. Until I found God, I did not know how to step outside of my false thoughts. At first when I was able to do so, it was brief. As I came to know God better and realized that when I was with Him I felt safe, I also realized I could actually stop my mind's scary thoughts. When my body shut down my immune system so it could give me the energy to run and save myself, it did not realize that it was my mind coming after me. The tiger chasing me was my *less than* mind, and the avalanche was the story I made up in my mind about what cancer was going to do to me. My anxiety about cancer was not serving me. Desperately trying to change the parts of cancer that were out of my control allowed fear to take hold. Letting go of my fear, the one thing I *could* control was one of the most healing things that knowing God and trusting His plan brought to me.

I'm not a doctor, and I know there are certainly many components to getting sick and being healed, but I can tell you that since I released the stress and fear from my *less than* thinking and fear of things out of my control by hanging out with God, I have not had so much as a cold.

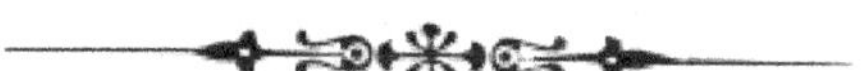

I learned during my sickness that God is amazing. I used to think I needed to have every detail worked out for both plan A and plan B. If anything was going to be done right, it would have to be done by me. When my mind was wiped out by the chemo, I could not even make a bad plan. Details were not something I could come up with. All I could do was leave the particulars in God's hands about how leaving the hospital was going to push death out of me. God has taught me that I can trust in Him and He will get me there. Wherever it is, however it needs to be.

A funny thing happens when death is in just about every thought that you and everyone else has when thinking about you. It crawls inside of you making you its host. It becomes a part of you. You feel it just as you feel your heart beat. It's in your breath and in your bones. It begins to seep from your sweat. Now I know how death smells. Worse yet, I know how it feels when it is attempting to take you out.

After I was admitted to the hospital for the third time, now on the cancer floor, my red blood count was very low. A healthy red blood cell count is twelve. When you get down to eight, they give you a transfusion. Mine was six. Red blood cells carry oxygen throughout your body. When there are not enough of them, your body does not have sufficient oxygen to function properly. This makes you extremely fatigued. You have a hard time breathing; some people turn blue. I was told that I needed a blood transfusion and was given a little brochure on some of the possible side effects. I was already again on powerful intravenous antibiotics for the MRSA making my first thought, *Here we go again, trying to plug up a hole that will probably cause what is left of the delicate structure of my now precarious dam to break*. With my less-than-stellar batting average with modern medicine, I decided that I did not need to be mixing someone else's problems with mine. What if *their* blood had cancer cells? Therefore, I, for once, decided to stop doubling down. My body was screaming for me to stop taking in everybody else's medicine. *For one damn second, please stop.* I told my shocked doctor that the blood transfusion risk/reward ratio was too high. Apparently, most people do not say no to this magic trick. He was not happy and shook his head. To assure him or that I was not trying to kill myself, I agreed that if my count fell any further or my breathing became too labored I would do the transfusion.

The doctor then ran a test on my remaining red blood cells to see if I had developed some sort of bone marrow problem or leukemia from the chemo that was causing my low red blood cell count. Fortunately, what was left of my red blood cell army was strong and passed that examination.

In addition to limited red blood cells, I only had a 300 white blood cell count. A normal white blood cell count is between 3,500 and 10,000. My immune system was almost nonexistent—which meant I was too.

I would not admit to anyone how tired I was. Just getting out of bed to go to the bathroom was so exhausting that I would take a nap afterward. I was doing everything in my power to not get a blood transfusion. So I would lie there, saving my sparse energy to pretend I was fine every time a doctor came in the room. I could not extend the same courtesy to the nurses.

When your body has been mercilessly battered by chemo and you are still pumping in more drugs, you start feeling its struggle to right the ship. The one thing I always felt after every chemo, surgery, or even needle poke was that my body wanted to live. It wanted to heal itself. I started feeling guilty for what I had done to my body. All it ever tried to do was keep me well, and I must say it held on longer than I had the right to expect. My body never gave up; never… not once. My mind deceived me, but my body was magnificent. I knew all it ever wanted to do was fix what was wrong. I knew my body was on my side; it always was. It never let me down. I let *it* down. I cried for what I had done to my body and what I was continuing to do to it.

Looking back, there was a clear trail of seemingly small health failings that had been mounting before I was diagnosed, but I had not been paying attention. I continuously had cysts pop up around my monthly cycle, which meant my hormones were out of balance. I was not sleeping soundly and was always tired. I started eating a steady diet of sugar to keep my energy up and had gained twenty pounds in two years. I was catching colds more frequently. My lymph nodes in my neck kept swelling. A couple of months before I was diagnosed, my liver hurt for a week. I also had bronchitis for the first time in my life a month before I was diagnosed.

Now, looking back, my body had been screaming for me to make changes, setting off the alarms, but my mind was busy tending other people's fires. My body was warning me; it did not want this to happen. Then who has to endure the brunt of my mind's actions? My body. "That is not fair," I apologized to my body over and over. Now, when I am not doing the best for it in some way, I try to remember how well it loyally served and stuck by me, even when I hadn't supported it.

Back then my mind was misdirected and unyielding. I was proud of its steadfastness and strength. This firm determination and unbreakable thinking caused my body to be battered over and over by life. Everything had to crash into my body again and again as my mind would not back down and let anything *less than* pass through. Life wasn't hard; my mind was. Life wasn't breaking me; my thoughts were. My subconscious *less than* mind would not acknowledge that my body was just flesh and would eventually crumble under the force of my *more than* shield's misperceived strength.

"Be still, and know I am God." Psalm 46:10

From the other side of the mirror looking out at myself, I now understood how the previous forty-plus years of fighting had left me a little more wounded every day. From behind the mirror, I knew cancer was just a reflection of my pain. My body knew it needed God; my mind did not want to listen. My body was falling apart under the guise of my mind hurting my heart and continuing to move me further away from my Truth. My body knew the space I had fallen into was now too wide and it could no longer bridge the distance of the chasm, trying to balance the lopsided thinking of my mind.

All I could really do was lie there in bed, day after day after day. I stayed in the hospital longer the third time than the first and second times because my body was in real trouble. I was too weak to even sit in a chair. So as I just lay there as the tests kept coming back, stating, "This marker is too high. This is function is too low."

I then started having electrical pains that ran up each side of my spine. They went from my lower back up to my neck. It felt like someone had put a live wire at the base of my spine and the electricity from it would make the muscles along the length my back bone spasm. I wanted to scream out when it happened, but I was too tired. I didn't know if it was happening because my body's electrical system was shorting out and shutting down or if it was trying to reboot itself. I told myself that, either way, it was going on—and there was nothing that I would do about it. I certainly would not tell the doctors; I knew that if I told the doctors they would run more tests or make me take more drugs. I had to sit there and let the shock waves roll their way up three or four times and then they would take a break. As painful as they were, I just sat there and let them make their way up my back, knowing once they made it to the top of my spine the pain would leave my body.

So when I could no longer move my mind or my body, I became more powerful. I could lessen my body's pain, without drugs, by just letting it pass through. I learned how to stop holding on to my pain, let it run its course, and leave my body, just by accepting it and being still enough to let it pass through.

When I was first diagnosed, I became obsessed with healing my body and then also started trying to figure out what was going on in my mind. When both my body and my brain gave out, it allowed me the opportunity to find what I really needed to do to heal myself; find my connection to God.

My mind was finally too tired to dictate all of its tyrannical demands to my body every minute of the day. This incapacity was well timed since my body was unable to comply anyway. I quickly learned the benefits of not just having stillness in my mind, but finding it in my body too. I had to, for the first time in decades, just sit in my body. This allowed me to begin sensing and being with my body again. My body was no longer just something outside of me used for carrying the groceries into the house. My mind and my body, now both exhausted, became equals. That dual stillness began to reset the balance. I relearned how to operate my mind and body on a more equitable footing with each other. My mind started acknowledging my body again. I could now listen to what my body was feeling and saying to me, not just my mind. The message I heard from my body was quite clear; it had veered too far off course and I was heading for a wall. That's when I knew that I needed something greater than what my mind and body had just found. I needed more if we were going to live. I needed to find something that was not *less than* and was not going to die. I needed what always was and what will always be. I needed to find the essence of life, which was God, within me.

When you are that far into your physical collapse, you have to reach across the chasm and create a sacred partnership with your inner voice of God *Over There.* You need to listen to the voice of life to hear how to live. I did not know how to do this. It just happened. All I remember doing was accepting that my condition was what it was and I, for the first time, was not trying to fix anything. At that point, I really had no choice since I could not think or move. I was just letting things be as they were, sitting with life not trying to run my life. It was then I noticed a voice. I did not know where it was coming from at first, as it was faint. I was not even sure if it was real, so I sat in the clear stillness of my mind and body and remained calm, to see if I could understand what it was saying. As I learned to hear it quietly speak in my mind, I found great comfort and I knew it was from a "for sure" place. At the time, I did not know it was my Truth; I just knew it was "for sure." It was a female voice of God that told me that I now needed to leave the hospital.

Of course, this was not a popular decision with the doctors, who viewed my idea as irrational. My mom was concerned too. I also was hesitant at first, as I remembered watching people on hospital drama shows pulling this stunt and thinking they were out of their minds, but the voice was unwavering and sure that it was time to go. The voice was also calmly reassuring that we would be all right if we did. Even though I was still too sick to get out of bed, I believed it, more than I ever believed any of my doctors. Deciding to listen to my voice and leave the hospital was the first time I ever stood in my Truth. Then I called it my "for sure" place. I had to find the strength in my heart to believe in something my mind could not see, putting my life on the line, trusting the voice knew more than I did about how to save my life. For a Type A personality that would research everything ten ways to Sunday before making a decision, this was an explosion, bringing down the wall between my mind and God. This is how I began to learn how to stand in my Truth, relaxing in my now quiet mind and still body, and opening my heart and trusting the voice of life, God.

I began to understand how to silence my mind and rely on God when I learned how to sit in peace within myself and accept life as it was given. I learned that my pain was not from what was happening but from how I dealt with it. From a place of fear, not love and peace. That's how I began to understand the power of God's presence and ability to change the energy of my illness. This was the beginning of changing my perception of sickness and health.

My friend Judy would always tell me to look inside my body and visualize a bright light emanating out of it. When I did that, I would somehow feel stronger, but I didn't really get how or why. It felt good, so I would do it whenever I remembered. Even though I had understood since sixth-grade science class that energy could neither be created nor destroyed but that its form could change, I just never considered that you could do this with the energy in your own body. But now I knew that when I was with God I could change the negative energy of fear and pain to peace. I still had many lessons to learn about how to implement this as a way of life, but this was my start.

Many months later, when I allowed myself to stand steadfastly in the place of Truth, I knew everything had changed. I now recalled that the night I was poked with all those needles for all those hours, I ran from *Here* and embraced the place *Over There.* When I was *Over There,* I could let the pain from what the doctors and nurses were doing to me move effortlessly through the stillness of my body. I knew I did this same trick with the shock waves moving up my spine. I had somehow learned how to be the gentle, clear stream, washing the event through, not the undercurrent cutting everything to pieces and recklessly littering my body with the residue. All the pain that I had held on to for so long now had been given the freedom to pass through and find its way out.

Now I know that when I learned to stay still, whatever was happening at that moment and needed to pass though had the freedom to do so. I finally learned that when you live in your Truth, you are standing still and everything can move through you. Nothing can harm you. It is the holding on that is unnatural. It is by allowing everything to pass through that you are able to experience peace. Once you find peace, you will know you are standing inside your Truth.

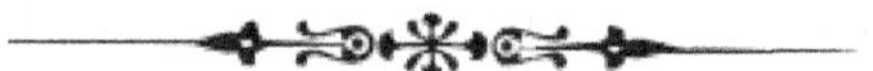

Choice is a most beautiful gift of love. You cannot acknowledge choice without trusting in the design. Knowing there is a choice brings a freedom to find the essence of the need. When something is chosen, it becomes celebrated. When something is chosen, it is valued and wholly owned. Choice has a sacred uniting force between the elector and the chosen.

The interesting thing is, once you are one with death, you understand it in ways that allow you to intuitively know what it needs in order to exist inside of you. The secret that I uncovered in the "for sure" knowing place inside of me is that to push out death, you must choose life. Everyone says they are choosing to live, but that is not the same as *choosing life*.

Sadly, I have seen many people in my cancer journey kid themselves about what they are actually choosing. I can spot them because I was one of them. Many people, even those who believe in God, become prisoners of their mind's thinking, and that keeps them from wholly being with God and His healing love. When I thought I was choosing to live, it was based on living from my mind. I was mired down in my human mind's thinking with its limited *less than* thoughts, judgments, fear, and unforgiveness that kept a wedge between me and God. I did not understand that choosing life and living through God, who is eternal life, was what would bring me enough love and peace to heal. Holding on to the familiar, subconscious, painful way of my mind's thinking and behavior seemed less uncomfortable than letting that go and holding on to God to live through His eternal life. I had to get out of my mean, controlling mind and open myself up to be one with God's love in order to create the greatest possibility of healing. I learned that choosing life means living outside my fearful mind and through the eternal part of me that is a part of God.

The choice to release everything on the way to the hospital was the first honest choice I had made for life in my life. Honestly and completely letting everything go and handing it to God allowed me to begin finding the way to stand in my Truth with God, outside of my mind's thoughts. The choice to listen to God's voice was my second critical choice. Trusting in God's voice is how I found the strength to get up out of that hospital bed and walk, albeit very slowly, out of that hospital. Staying there was only allowing death's grip to tighten around me.

My third and most important choice was the choice for life—not just *to live.* Understanding how to remain outside of my mind and *always* choosing to live though God was still a choice I was unable to make most days, but I did make it that day! How any of these choices were going to push death out of me, I had no idea.

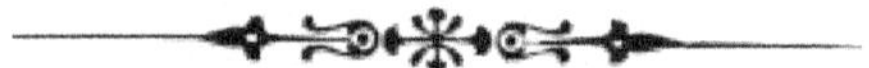

The greatest transformation happens when you realize that who you really and eternally are is Truth. Truth never alters but stands as it is, regardless of whatever is passing through. Everything that happens Here is only just a moment in time. Any given moment and everything within it is continuously changing, but only passing through your Truth. It is your choice to attack life's moments and try to make them more, less, or different than what they are: something passing through. When you embrace who you are, Truth, and live from there, everything can move through you as it is given.

"This is the day for which the LORD hath made; we will rejoice and be glad in it." Psalm 118:24

Aside from the female voice of God, Dan was my only other ally in my campaign to leave the hospital. He came to cautiously claim what was left of me, and I somehow found the will to hold on to him and leave the hospital. I was told that I was not well enough to leave. I needed to stay. I needed more tests. I needed more red blood cells.

I needed more white blood cells. I needed more medicine. I knew how sick I was, and after a week in the hospital, I knew I wasn't getting better. I also knew what the doctors could not see in my chart: I needed to leave or I would die.

As we began the 90-mile drive home from the hospital, I sat, quietly hunched over in the front passenger seat of our minivan, trying to act less sick than I really was. I was tired, in pain, and too nauseated to sit up straight. About thirty minutes into the ride, I heard a song I liked on the radio. Then it happened. I whispered a word from the song. I then found the strength to softly murmur a line from the song, which generated a giant lump in my throat. I was so touched by the emotion rising in me that tears started streaming down my face as I mumbled more words over the lump in my throat. I could not stop crying because I somehow now understood. I now realized that the only thing I had been given for sure, no take-backs, was this very moment to sing this song and be with my husband in the front seat of our minivan. I was not offered, nor did I want or think about, any other thing. This had never happened before in my demanding, hurry-up world. I felt at great peace, happy, and alive. I understood in that knowing, "for sure" place inside me there was no death in that beautiful moment that I had been given.

That moment, I would find out later, I had experienced from my Truth. Hunched over, mumbling, crying, and accepting life only as it was given. Unconditionally loving that moment with all its glory and limitations and not requiring any more from it than it had to give. I really, for the first time in all my life, realized what it was like to be truly alive; in that moment, living right now. Time had stopped and I was only inside of my Truth with God, inside of my eternity *Over There*, simultaneously accepting, embracing, and dancing with what life was offering me *Here*. It was God taking me to my Truth and allowing me to experience, for the first time, the real and honest miracle of life *Here* that pushed out the death that had crept within me. I'm glad I left the plan up to God. Not only did it work; it forever changed every moment, moving forward, that I would experience *Here* on Earth.

I had no idea how God worked. I learned in my Truth that even when I was sitting in the darkness of the chasm that I never really needed to figure out how I was going to get out. I only needed to trust in God and know that everything was going to work out just the way it would, just the way it should. There was only ever one light that needed to be seen, and that was God's. I only needed to continue to build my relationship with God and remain in faith that He would pave the way. I only had to understand that at that very moment, as I sat lost in the bleak chasm, God was stirring hearts, harmonizing destinies, and shaping circumstances, to align and light my passageway to *Over There.*

After I returned home, I was still weak and sick. My body was still fighting the MRSA and I was taking strong antibiotics. Due to my low blood cell counts, I was exhausted, and if I walked, my low potassium levels caused my heart to convulse and pound so hard I thought it was going to explode out of my chest. This was all going on in addition to still being heavily under the influence of the chemo side effects. I didn't talk much due to my fatigue and nausea, but when I did, I kept hearing myself tell people, "God cured me." The words just kept falling out of my mouth. I kept telling people, "The chemo almost killed me, but God cured me." Whenever I said it, I was taken aback since I really never talked about God before and now my first words about Him, and the only thing that kept coming from my mouth, was how God healed me. I could not stop myself from saying it at that point, though, since the chemo took away my brain's mental capacity to filter anything I was thinking or saying. Later in my pilgrimage, when the female voice of God told me that I could trust the words that fall out of my mouth before I could catch them, I recalled my words about God healing me.

PART 5

Learning My Truth

I know that when I was at my sickest I had no choice but to be open to any possible information that may have helped save my life. Once I realized that chemo cures less people than it saves, I knew I needed a better game plan than the doctors were offering if I wanted to live. I knew I needed to find my way outside of medicine's box and embrace something bigger if I was going to continue my life.

Everyone would tell me, "Don't claim your cancer. Don't say, '*My* cancer.' Everyone who says, '*My* cancer' gets it back and dies." I understood that when people made their illness part of their identity and found some sort of emotional payoff from it, they were most likely not going to recover, but that was not what my words were doing. I also understood the power of words and respected that you should not call things to you that you do not want. Therefore, I would let their words go, but I always felt annoyed every time someone would say that to me. I am disciplined and, as a sales consultant, knew how to carefully pick my words for a living, so I knew how to *stop* using words that did not serve me. Nevertheless, I kept hearing myself saying it: "*My* cancer."

Since my *less than* mind always blamed me when things went wrong in my life, I never freaked out and blamed the outside world for giving me cancer. I never said, "Who did this to me? Why me?" Although it came out of left field and my ideas about life did not include cancer, I did not see a flag on the play. I did not feel a need to lodge a protest about getting cancer. Even later when I would learn about pesticides, GMOs, hormones and antibiotics in meat, xenoestrogens, white sugar, trans fats, high-fructose corn syrup, prescription medications, electromagnetic waves and radiation from wireless devices, root canals, and fluoride, I recognized that those things may have been a part of creating an environment for cancer, but I still felt that my mind's stress had been the greater part of *my* cancer.

I also never blamed God. I instinctively ran to God immediately. Maybe not in the most appropriate or graceful way, but I intuitively believed enough to try to reach Him. I didn't get mad at Him. I am grateful that I chose to become soft toward God when things were becoming very hard.

After a dreadful two months of battling someone else's cancer, I again said, "*My* cancer" to someone I was talking to on the phone and was once more warned of the error of my words. Now, lots of words came to me about, "*My* cancer." If it is not mine and it's yours, then take it back. If it's not mine and it's not yours, should I put it in the lost-and-found? Where did it come from anyway? Did an alien put it in my body? I just said, "Okay, whose cancer is it? Really?" I made an excuse and got off the phone.

I immediately said to myself, "I think maybe it's time I stand up and admit that it's mine. "Hi, my name is Carol Ulrich and I 'claim' this cancer as mine. It is *my* cancer!" It felt liberating to say that. I didn't hear the usual foreboding "*Dant-dant-da!*" after claiming *my* cancer.

The truth is, I hadn't really claimed anything about myself in a really long time. I side-stepped ownership and responsibility of myself because my mind had me busy claiming other people's care, needs, wants, business, and any other thing outside of myself I found along the way. That day, I claimed *my* cancer. I also claimed *my*self again and began to understand that fixing *my* cancer was more than just doing chemo. It was about healing the parts of *my*self that allowed it to be created. I had no idea how I was going to do it though.

I began to feel that the space for cancer to grow inside of me was formed because I had let go of too many things I should have kept inside of me. I let my life force get low. I gave away too much, always trying to be better than what my mind told me I was. I pushed through and did more, trying not to be *less than* one too many times, and then cancer pushed through me. I ignored my body's cues that it was growing weak. I let my candle burn too low, and a small whiff of air was able to blow it out. I played such a deceptive shell game with myself, constantly moving those cups around, mistakenly thinking I knew where the ball was. Then I lost track of my center, and one day, when I lifted *my* cup it was empty.

So there it is. I did it. It was mine. It does not matter that my subconscious, mean, *less than* mind caused me to do it. It only matters that I found an awareness and acknowledged that it happened from inside of me so that I could claim my choice to change *my* mind. I found that you can always make a new choice about yourself, for yourself.

When I became sick, I had no idea what my beliefs were that made me act the way I did. I had always thought and acted like that. I just assumed I was me being me. I had no idea that I could be another way in the world. I also had no idea God was the solution to my mind's constant barrage of judgments against myself and others. At that time, I believed my subconscious mind that told me I was separate from everyone, including God. I also believed that I was *less than*, as I judged myself all day, every day. The stress of these unknown beliefs made me always do too much, in order to be *more than*, and always feel hurt by others' actions, perceiving them as a direct attack for me being *less than*.

The subconscious negative mind, or the ego, uses your false beliefs to stay in charge and keep running your life. It is the part of your mind that hyper-defends itself and over-reaches reality, creating false thoughts that cause you fear and insecurity. It does this by telling you that you are separate from everyone, including God. It convinces you of your separateness by constantly telling you that you are *less than* others in some way. It is always trying to convince you that you need to continue to attempt to make yourself *more than*. The subconscious mind then has you trapped in its stress and chaos of trying to fix yourself and others so you can stop being *less than*. You are too busy fighting the world alone and not being good enough to remember that there is another voice inside of you. The voice of God will tell you that you are not alone and your *less than* beliefs are false. God's voice lovingly tells you that you are already enough.

For me, my subconscious thoughts and feelings led to emotional stress and behaviors that consequently harmed my body. When I worried excessively about my kids and job, and always thought I needed to do more to be better, I created real physical effects from the emotions of those thoughts. My blood pressure would go up, my heart would beat faster, and I would get anxious. That stress was a real physical thing emanating from the thoughts in my mind, and it did real biological harm to my body, including my cells.

Those thoughts also led to other behaviors. I did not find the time to exercise or eat healthfully because I always had to be more and better for someone else. I ate way too much sugar to make sure I could keep up an unrealistic daily pace. I wasn't able to sleep, thinking and worrying about everything and anything. All of these behaviors caused even more physical damage to my body and my cells. My mind's unloving thoughts had placed unrealistic obligations on my body, causing damage that it could not sustain.

Did I do it purposefully? No; I was doing the best I could, based on the subconscious thoughts I had believed in my mind about myself and this world since I was a child. It was still a few months away, when I fell even further, that I realized the weakness in my mind's thinking. Even then, understanding how to change my mind from a level beneath those thoughts was elusive. At this point in time, I had no idea about what was going on in my head and was too sick to figure it out.

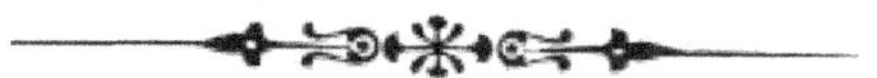

Some doctors, researchers, and spiritualists say you get sick or in an accident because you want to die. I don't think I wanted to die, although, I may have wanted a way out of the pain my mind had created. Unwilling to acknowledge this, other than through a bag of Doritos and some chocolate-chip cookie dough, it took cancer to bring me to the point where I had to change or I would die. My mean mind created my worst nightmare. The thing that is interesting to me now—though not then—is how cancer came and how it unfolded revealed everything I needed to know about myself in order to find God.

Does everyone who has cancer, another disease, or something else bad happen to them choose it? No, of course not. Everyone has their own path and their own story. However, I do believe everyone's story is a combination of circumstances and events that create it. Some people may have had something enter their body that caused it to break down or it may have already been there in their DNA. Other people may have experienced too much hardship or maybe life's lottery just pick their name. Even though everything that causes a disease may not be within someone's control, I believe everyone can have hope for healing because there are always aspects of people's stories that they can actually change. I believe my cancer had several components, but the biggest factor was the way I had lived my life without God. This allowed my mind to inflict too much pain into my heart, suppressing my immune system and leaving my body vulnerable to breaking down.

At first I didn't think the cancer was from my mind or that it was even in the realm of possibility. I certainly did not say it out loud or with the certainty that I do now. In the beginning when the idea that it might be possible surfaced in my research, I was open to considering it just like any other test or examination I had. All I was interested in was finding healing regardless of where it came from. I decided that when you are sick you can deflect and defend or you can be profoundly honest and open to any possibility of healing.

Everyone's story is a personal covenant between them and God. No one is capable of understanding or knowing about anyone else's Truth, which may include why or how they need to leave or stay in this world. I knew I needed to fix my mind to heal my cancer. I just didn't know how.

It is the destination, not the journey. I was on and off what I believed to be the spiritual journey for years but never plugged a destination into the GPS.

I wanted to be calm and happy, but I didn't know what to do to achieve that. Everyone kept saying, "It's the journey, not the destination," so I never planned on ending up anywhere in particular. I spent my life *Here* running around, on a circular track, misguidedly doing an erroneous high school algebra equation. I painstakingly calculated how many apples I could load into my train while circling the station at top speed, all the while wanting everyone see how much smoke was blowing out of my train's engine. I never figured out the answer based on following any particular tracks or steering toward any necessary crossings. It never even occurred to me to pay attention to the lighted signs that would have lovingly pointed me to my destination, because I didn't know I was supposed to end up somewhere. So I chugged, at break-neck speed, through my days with the subject of answering life's questions at the bottom of my to-do list. I thought the floundering and seeking were what would take me to where I wanted to be, so that's exactly what I did. Why didn't anyone tell me my train was running out of steam and I needed to get back to a place I had forgotten? Why wasn't I figuring out how to get *Over There* instead of inhaling toxic smoke and sitting in now rotten apples *Here*?

I now know you need to be seeking the destination, your Truth that resides in God: the only place where peace resides. When you get so sick that you can hear the clock ticking every second, the haunting chimes every fifteen minutes, and know that big bongs are coming every hour, you need to ditch the algebra and buy a one-way ticket on the express to your destination so you can stand on the solid ground of Truth ahead of the grim reaper.

There is no place better than the fertile land of Truth to release your fear, allowing you to find enough peace and love to heal; where time is timeless and you know there will be a tomorrow. *Over There* allows you to find enough love for yourself to choose life. I didn't know how to get there, or how long it would take, but that is where I needed to be. Because there lay the secret of life, happiness, and health.

The truth of Truth is that only you can know your Truth. No one else can know your Truth for you.

When I arrived on the cancer floor in Fargo for my third hospitalization with MRSA, a thousand miles from the cancer hospital in Chicago, a new oncologist came to my room to oversee my care. As she was examining my right breast, I asked her if the tumor was growing back. She laughed as she pressed harder on my breast. Not feeling anything, she said, "Tumors don't grow back in a few weeks." The oncologist then said, through her laughing smile at my question, "That's not the way cancer works." What I did know was that three doctors and one physician's assistant had not felt my tumor for over a month at that point. I also I knew that since the chemo eliminated my tumor there was only a ten percent chance of reoccurrence later on, so I wasn't sure why I would have thought about it coming back after a few weeks, or why I even brought it up. At that point I felt the doctor had to know more about cancer than me and probably had treated thousands of other cancer patients so I should believe her. I decided that my thought that it was going to grow back was born from my unexpected bouts of MRSA. Even so, I felt embarrassed about my feelings. I decided that I had asked because I was still outrunning fear.

I did not bring it up again, telling myself it was a silly, paranoid thought. I tried to convince myself that the truth was in her words. Having exiled my intuition, I certainly was not thinking I had any particular affinity for determining truth. At that time, I didn't even know that it was possible to know your Truth. I took anyone's version of the truth and accepted it in any manner it was delivered, never trusting how it felt inside of me. Truth at that point lived outside of me in whatever form it was given.

Three weeks later I was out of the hospital and was preparing to go to Chicago to discuss my lumpectomy surgery. I was feeling better, as if I had it all under control again. Like a hero winning again and making it through the storm—overcoming adversity, taking control, and being triumphant. No signs of a tumor. No signs of MRSA. I told my mom she could go home thinking that I was good to go. I was actually excited to go to Chicago with good news. I would go there powerful, tightly holding up my *more than* shield, touting my victory over death. My shield that I was now using to protect myself from my *less than* mind reminding me that it was my fault for almost dying because I got cancer in the first place. This moment was something I had dreamt about: going back, not as just a rock star but a Grammy winner. I wanted to be like the survivors with good news that I had met in the limo, able to cheer on the others. I thought I was on the downside of the mountain of this journey.

Then my breast started hurting a little. I told myself that I was being paranoid and that it didn't mean anything. *I'm sure it's normal.* I felt around anyway: nothing there, just like the doctor said. The next day it hurt a little more, and more often. I didn't want to check for a lump again. I had just done that the day before and I didn't feel anything. I thought I was being ridiculous to think something was happening, but the sharp throbs of pain finally caused me to try to soothe my breast with my hand, and there it was—a lump. By the following day, the day before I was to leave, the lump had turned into an orange inside my breast. I couldn't believe it; the tumor *had* come back. I was told this didn't happen. I was told that cancer did not work that way. I was laughed at.

What I had known that day in the hospital when I asked if the tumor had grown back was the real Truth of my breast cancer. I had known the truth from my Truth and denied it, accepting that doctor's untruths about my breast cancer tumor and regrowth.

I have rewritten the memory of this conversation not just for me, but also for others to find it in the Truth when they need it. I now have that oncologist in the hospital say to me, "Carol, because you asked if your tumor may grow back, I think you may have become aware of your Truth and sense it as I cannot. This is just the beginning for you really knowing yourself and God. This means you are now on the path to learning how to heal yourself. So even if the tumor does grow back, know that it is a sign that you now can acknowledge your Truth. This understanding of Truth will ultimately set you free from cancer. This is a special day for you—a turning point in your healing. I am blessed to have witnessed it. God bless your awakening."

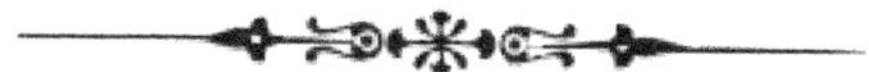

Possibility is not probability or plausibility. It is only acknowledging the belief that you can experience the Truth of something other than what you know at this moment. Possibility is believing in the unseen, the potential of something other than what is currently revealed at this time. If you were new to this planet and knew nothing about the germination process of plants, would you believe that a seed could grow into a magnificent flower? You might say that you believe in the possibility even though you do not know how, since you have not seen plants grow. The next thing I would hope you would say is that you made that presumption because you believe that anything is possible.

My most precious son Daniel, now eleven years old, has come home from school many times over his academic career with multiple-choice worksheets and test answers marked as "wrong." The questions usually have one theme: seeking his conclusion as to what was needed to make something happen or what occurred after a certain scenario happened. Many times he circles, "All of the above." When we look at the worksheet or test and I review the questions that are marked "wrong," Daniel's enthusiastic explanation is always that all of the scenarios are possible. He excitedly says, "Mom, anything is possible—right?" Daniel's brilliance resides in the knowing that his heart tells him that although some of the answers are more palatable based on the current evidence, the other answers should not be disregarded or treated with less dignity than the obvious answer. He will not ignore the fact that they are all possible. I have never and will never tell him that he is wrong about his decision to circle "All of the above." He is beautifully, simply right. He has taught me more about Truth than my law degree could even conceive. God brought this message of belief to me through my son. That is how I know all things are possible.

As I waited for my flight from Minneapolis to Chicago to now talk about my tumor regrowth, I was shaking in fear. It was uncontrollable. I was in full panic. I tried to call my friend Judy three times as I sat in an empty row of chairs at Minneapolis Airport. The first two attempts, I could not stop my fingers from shaking long enough to touch the right contact number on the phone's screen. The third time I got lucky. Even though my fingers and hands would not stop shaking, the time between the movements of my right hand's fingers and the location of Judy's number on the phone in my unsteady left hand somehow matched up and the call went through. I was grateful she answered, and I desperately cried as I told her what had happened. As we were speaking, my hands would still not stop trembling, and the merciless fear in my fingers was constantly threatening to hang up on my lifeline. Although I found a way to hold on and stay connected to Judy through my shaking and tears, I still needed to find a way to hold on and stay connected with what would ultimately save me: God.

Through my feverish hysteria of tears, I told her I needed a miracle. I begged her to tell me if she knew of anyone who had had a miracle happen to them. She told me about a guy who had a stroke and could not speak for a year until he started taking a new medication and then he began talking again. She thought that could be considered a miracle. I knew that was not a big enough miracle for my situation, though, especially the medicine part. However, what *was* big enough was when she told me that miracles are always possible and that if anyone could expect one, it should be me. She did not waver on the prospect of a miracle for me, and I started holding on more steadily to the possibility also. At that moment, I believed more in the possibility than the impossibility.

After I arrived in Chicago and before my mom arrived to be with me in my moment of uncertainty, I sat in my hotel room, exhausted, quiet, and contemplative about what was happening to me. Long tears rolled down my cheeks as I asked the pounding questions in my head. "How could I have healed and backtracked so far as to have a lump in my breast four times bigger than when I started chemo three months earlier?" I heard the oncologist's words again: "That's not how cancer works." Then I got frustrated and confoundedly wondered, "What happened to make cancer work this way on me? Why was cancer so hard on me? Why did everything keep going wrong? Why was it that winning was fleeting and always meant more losing was ahead?"

I thought about the fact that I never lost anything that I really wanted and went after, regardless of the difficulty and sacrifice of getting it. I could not understand why I was losing now if living was what I needed more than anything I ever wanted. I had fought for everything my whole life, trying to be good enough, but had never had to fight *this* hard. Now my human strength could not give me what I needed to live. My must have win was going to be my most devastating defeat. I sat in disbelief, thinking that of all the things to start a losing streak with, cancer was the one that would cost me my life. I then asked the right question: "Why was it that just when I was gaining my physical and mental strength back, it exposed a greater weakness?"

The regrowth was the most unbelievable physical thing that had happened to me thus far. Even more incredible was the fact that I still didn't fully understand that I wasn't just in an accident; I *created* the accident. I still did not recognize that holding up my subconscious *more than* shield every day, trying to protect myself from my subconscious mean mind's attacks, was done as I stood in front of oncoming traffic. What I did know was that this was my third strike, and I was pretty sure I was out. This vengeful reemergence of my tumor represented a sad, discernible pattern of *my* cancer journey. This orange in my breast made me look at myself and know that my best efforts and the strengths I always used to win were leading to a permanent loss this time. My way of being in the world and winning at life *Here* seemed to be my downfall when it came to cancer. I desperately wanted to change but didn't know how or what would make a difference at that point.

Sitting on the edge of the bed, I was not at my worst physically. It had been two weeks since I left the hospital, and I was doing okay. The other times when I had been on the ropes with chemo and MRSA, I knew that I could die, but my mind and body were so weak that I could only churn the foggy pieces of the possibility of death. This time I was fully cognizant of my mortality. I had death staring at me, and I was clearly looking at its orange-sized form front and center in my breast. I was able to fully feel the reality of dying for the first time. That's when I wholeheartedly admitted to myself that living may not be my end game with cancer. I knew about the fact that when triple-negative returns, it's just a matter of time. It's not *if* you are going to live but *how much longer* you would live. I had to consider that there was a strong possibility that what was going on in my breast was now going on in the rest of my body. It's not that I didn't want to live, but I needed to yield to the fact that the odds of doing so were now much more limited. I needed to move my mind's laser focus from fighting against being a *less than* with cancer to accepting in my heart that it might be time to end the battle and to call a truce. I was not going to squander what was left of my time here in a death match struggle. After reflecting on the fact that I had no idea what to do or how to do anything differently, I decided to stop thinking about it for now. I drifted off to sleep for forty-five minutes or so and then my mom arrived.

It was now late and I showed her my new lump and cried some more. She did not say what she thought it meant. Mom was concerned but not hysterical like me. My mom brought her love to me. She put her lifeline around me and made me feel like I would be kept from falling as long as she could hold on to me. I knew she had great strength but what was happening to me was too heavy to be held by anyone. It was then that I realized that the strength of everything about me made me hard to save. I was too much. I used to pride myself on being the strongest, the most immovable—someone whom people could not take down. Who can save that person? I didn't realize that the same tactics your mind uses to keep people and life from hurting you are the exact same things that *keep* people and life from helping you. All I knew then was that I couldn't even bear the weight of my being. This made letting go not only necessary but really my only choice. It did not feel like a choice at that moment, as it came naturally and with a sense of relief. It actually felt a bit peaceful to drop my strong, immovable *more than shield* that took all my strength to hold up all day, every day, so I wouldn't feel *less than*—even if it was only in that moment, to sit quietly in the space of my chasm.

After I was all cried out, I chose to open my heart and fully believe in miracles. I had now experienced enough of God and was able to trust in the love God had shown me. Right before I fell asleep, and even though I knew it was a long shot, I humbly asked God for a miracle. My mind was exhausted, and I was again on my knees with nowhere else to turn, allowing me to escape my thoughts and truly open my heart with my unconditional request. I told God my love of Him was complete and would not waver, even without the miracle. I sat deep in my Truth without fear and found myself not requiring any more than what would be given to me. I was at peace with myself and with God. This was the first time I sat wholly in my Truth and honestly, from the peace of Truth, accepted that living might not be my outcome with cancer. Even though I wanted so badly to live, I let go of that requirement from God. I was no longer going to let my mind bark orders about my life, type up a list of demands, and hold me and everyone else, including God, hostage until I was good enough. This was the space in which I wholeheartedly acknowledged my faith. I somehow learned to love and trust God unconditionally and sit peacefully with Him in the space of not knowing. It was the second time I gave it all over to God. In the minivan on the way to the hospital, it was my heart pausing to offer me a moment to open up to God before I died that had brought Him to me, but now I did it steadfastly from within my Truth; from somewhere deep and trusting that understood what I had not all along.

Now looking back, I realize that as my strength returned after my fourth chemo and MRSA, my stressful mind forced me to lift my old familiar shield of protection from being *less than*. All of those false beliefs sat there along with the orange in my breast. It was that thinking that sapped my real strength and again stopped the flow of my true power, God, what I really needed to heal me. What I sought out of mental and physical force to provide me with security from my mind was my downfall. My power came when I laid down my shield and stopped listening to my *less than* mind. I realize now that if I had known the strength of staying with God, not just when I was knocked down but after I was again able to stand up, I could have healed. I would have understood that with God I was more than enough as I stood. There was no need to strain every minute of the day holding up a shield of false bravado to protect me from my *less than* mind. It may now be obvious to you that trusting in my own strength should have made me fearful, but back then I didn't understand that my subconscious and unknown mind's *less than* thoughts continuously pelted me, which made it necessary to use a shield to protect myself.

My story is about learning that there is another way. In my most desperate times, when the pain was too much and I had nowhere else to turn, I reached out to God. Even though it was a long shot and I did not feel worthy, He came. However, most days when I was still distressed but wasn't facing imminent extinction, my mind told me that I did not have the right to be with Him. It took me a while, but I learned that when I called God would answer. I thought calling on God was like ordering pizza. I would pick up the phone, ask for help, and maybe it would be delivered—hopefully in thirty minutes or less. I didn't know that you didn't have to be starving for Him before you tried to reach him. I thought God was down the street. I didn't know God was already inside of me. I just didn't understand that my *less than* mind is what severed the connection.

I didn't know it was possible to be with God all the time for comfort and strength. My mind had me believe that it would provide me with that, but all it ever did was make me feel separate from God and *less than* everyone else. I never realized that I dropped my connection to God the second I listened to my *less than* mind and lifted my shield. I had not yet realized that when I laid down my *more than* shield and opened my heart to God, He would always provide love, protection, and healing from my mind.

Rejoining God occurs naturally when you lay down your false mind. But until you can step outside of your false thoughts, you painfully think that believing in God means you are only losing your importance and self-control.

The way I learned to remain with God was by staying outside of my subconscious negative mind. As long as you do not feel separate and you know you are *more than* enough just as you are, the negative mind can be quieted and you can be with God.

Before I was sick, I would watch this spider weaving her web every day as I made several trips in and out of my garage. I pondered if she ever tired of spinning that web day after day. For some reason I would only knock down her web when she was not in it. Every time I did so I wondered if she got mad, knowing that she would have to reweave her safety net. I decided that I would not like being a spider; every time you need to rest, or have to leave your web to try to do something for yourself, you have to hope your protective shelter was not destroyed as you were doing so. The instant you know it remains intact, you then have to question, "Did the web catch something more for me? Did my hard work yield me a victory to make it through another day?" I knew I did not want to be a spider.

It turned out my web was much more complex than the spider's. I spent so many years weaving a web around my mind's thoughts to make me feel secure. Day in and day out I worked on my safety net, jumping out of bed to take care of everything: the kids, the house, and my job. At night after dinner, dishes, showers, and everything else, I would sigh right before going to bed and think, I made it through another day, intact. The funny thing about the word "life" is that when you take out one letter it becomes a lie! A perfect web—a perfect trap. Look what I caught: cancer.

I soon learned that the spider did not want to be me either. She knew more than I did. She knew her web was not built for safety. It was only made for however long it lasted. She did not fear her web being knocked down by me or anyone else, because she knew building and rebuilding her web was all that life *Here* had to offer.

I'm not saying that everyone's mind alone can either create or cure all that ails them. All I am saying is that I realized that I needed to include being more mindful of my thoughts and emotions as part of my healing formula. I needed to heal the part of my mind that contributed to the stress in my body, which played its part in weakening my immune system and allowed cancer to grow. I was able to understand this about myself because I remembered feeling bad enough about the weight of these kinds of thoughts to go to a therapist a few years after my second son was born. I had never gone to therapy before, but I was exhausted from not being able to sleep at night and thought it would help me relax my mind enough to rest. Although getting a full night's sleep was my main goal, I was also secretly hoping that I could figure out how to stop feeling guilty and not good enough when I was awake; both at work and when I was at home. My full-time, pressured filled job along with the demands of caring for two small children lessened my ability to hold my subconscious, mean mind's judgements of my lacking at bay. I was in a constant battle against two opposing forces of never being good enough: career woman and motherhood. This was a battle for my time and energy that created an insurmountable level of guilt and stress that I had never had to contend with before. It was also a fight that I was never going to win until I found God.

While I was trying to find my living will paperwork for the hospital, I found my therapy goals from my initial meeting with a therapist years prior. Of course, being a Type A personality, I had a list of typed-up objectives. Now having cancer, what I found was no longer a mere outline of missed targets from the past but a directive that would be my roadmap to healing.

Top Goals of Therapy

1. I want to stop working so hard to get approval/love both awake and asleep. I want to just show up and be/feel enough "as is."

2. I want to stop being so hard on myself—so judgmental of myself. I want my first response and thoughts about myself to be loving, comforting, compassionate, and not so critically serious all the time. I want to treat myself the way I am with my kids.

3. I do not want to feel as if I always have to protect myself and everyone around me. I don't want to have to control/plan/execute everything to feel safe.

I did not cure anything then. I only went for a month. I put on my salesman's game face and enthusiastically did whatever the therapist asked, but it ended up being too small a deal to earn a commission. She said I had a lot of positive energy but never noticed my heart was broken. She told me to forgive people but never told me how to stop being hurt by people. She said to not work so hard but didn't tell me why I thought I should. Maybe the therapy didn't stick because she never mentioned God.

I just wanted to take a breath. I wanted to sit down and relax. I didn't want to always feel like I should be doing more and that it would never be enough. I wanted a moment to be still. But I didn't know how. The therapist was sure I was fine telling me that I was just experiencing "life's stress" with young children and that there was nothing really to *fix*. So I left thinking everyone *Here* felt like I did and that I would just have to deal with those feelings like everyone else. Of course thinking they somehow managed to do so better than me. So I pushed those thoughts down until the chatter again became inaudible. But the stress I felt every time I was at the doctor's office or school event with my kids instead of being at work or on a business trip and not at home with my kids was always there. Cancer turned up the volume on these thoughts and I began to hear what my subconscious mind had been shouting but I had managed to keep the mute button on for over forty years. Cancer required me to take the time to meet my goal with a mandated expiration time stamp on it. Now I really had to find the "cure" for all that ailed me, not just the cancer.

Several months after my cancer treatment was complete, I figured out that people's *less than* minds cause them to do some combination of withdrawing, attacking, or deflecting of life in varying degrees of intensity. People may withdraw by hiding under the influence of something to avoid and distract them from their subconscious mind's accusations of imperfectness, incompleteness, or unlovableness. This numbing ritual can be done in a multitude of ways, allowing the person to forget about their mind's judgments of their lacking. Everyone knows the rituals of doing anything too much, including alcohol, drugs, food, work, gambling, the Internet, etc. Many say they are doing these things to relax from their stressful lives but never see that the greater part of their stressful life comes from their subconscious mind's constant barrage of negative fearful thoughts. If they could quiet their minds and connect with God, they would find their stressful life much more peaceful.

Other people are more aggressive in fighting what they are hearing from their subconscious mind. Since they do not know how to defend themselves from their mind's judgments, they instead choose to defend themselves from what their mind tells them about other people's judgments. This approach follows the "get them before they get me" philosophy. They will attack everyone, using swords like egotism, hostility, control, or physical violence. They hear all day, every day how much they are *less than* from their minds and will not take the chance on letting anyone else chime in.

Although I could certainly withdraw or attack, I most strongly aligned with the deflect group: the group of people who use themselves as human shields to repel the hurt being inflicted by their *less than* minds. These folks may offer up their lives and time to others by being people pleasers or doormats in order to try to deflect their subconscious pronouncements. They may also fend off the pain of not being good enough by hiding underneath the underachiever shield so others cannot judge them for being a failure like their mind already has done. I tightly held up the overachiever shield. The shield made out of my accomplishments, tightly bound together yet never strong enough. This left me always trying to be more and better so I could fend off other people's judgments of my lacking. Unfortunately, I didn't realize that the judgments of others that I feared were coming from the same place as my judgments—our *less than* minds.

I finally uncovered my long-running subconscious story: I always had to earn my acceptance from others. This meant doing more than everyone else did so no one would be able to reject me. It's amazing how your mind can easily take something small and twist your thoughts around it for years until it runs your life off the tracks. My false belief was formed easily enough when I was younger and a few kids would always exclude me from playing with them, telling me I wasn't welcome, making me feel unworthy and not good enough. This rejection was hurtful. My seven-year-old self's solution and behavior going forward, in order to avoid experiencing that hurt again, had been to create an overachiever shield. Carrying a *more than* shield to protect me from any future rejection meant that I had to try harder and do more. I had to earn every drop of worthiness in advance so that people would have to accept me. No one would be able to reject me again by saying I wasn't good enough. If I were better than them they would have no choice but to play with me. If they still chose to exclude me, I could walk away telling myself that it was not because I was *less than* them, diminishing the hurt from their rejection. I worked overtime trying to be more entertaining, stronger, smarter, and more successful than others. I had to have more *more thans* than others did. That way when my mean mind would remind me of my seven-year-old self's rejection, I could lift my *more than* shield and protect myself from the memory of the hurt. I would be safeguarded from it happening again.

I believed that acceptance was something that would never be given to me. I had to earn it. Looking back, was it true? Sometimes I remembered people who had made me earn my place; that's life. However, with most of my experiences, which didn't require earning acceptance, my mind filled in the blanks and my expectation was always that I would need to put extra effort into everything to be good enough. I always worked much harder at accomplishing things than I needed to, thinking that was the only way to earn them.

I now believe that the same success would have come to me even if I didn't work overtime, every time, trying to get it. I pushed so hard that I chased things rather than let them come to me in the natural course of my endeavors. I was paddling my boat so hard upstream that the wake sent a wave toward whatever I wanted and pushed it further away from me. So I would paddle harder and harder against the current, eventually getting enough exertion into my strokes to beat the counterforce I had created. I would never let anything go. I was beyond proactive. I was a non-stop ball of undisciplined energy moving the force of life's gifts further away from me, and whenever that happened I would then really get going. I made things much more difficult for myself. Life did not do that to me… *I* did. My mind did that with everything, including cancer.

Maybe if I had decided that I was good enough just to make the required effort, not a hyper effort. If I had understood that my positive personally, what I had learned in school and in the world, along with my natural abilities, and solid work ethic was enough, I could have paddled my boat with confident, knowing strokes. This would have provided the right balance to hold it steady in the current. Then life's gifts that were coming to me through the natural flow of my efforts would have arrived and I could have simply reached out and picked up what was mine. It wasn't until I stopped trying to chase healing that healing came to me over and over. Then, sure enough, as soon as I got stronger I would jump in, start stirring the water, and cause another tidal wave that again threatened my life. *Seriously?* I needed someone to grab me by the shoulders, hold me still and lovingly say, "For Pete's sake, stop this madness. It does not have to be like this. You are good enough." And someone did: God.

I think it is lyrical how God, who is love, wholeness, and perfection, resides inside human beings who believe they are anything *but* loved, complete, and enough. How amazing is it that right next to the mind's thinking about unlovingness, singularity, and *less than* is the Truth, which is the exact opposite?

I went back and talked to myself as a seven-year-old little girl. First I hugged me because I was so cute. Then I kissed my cheek because I was so innocent. I told that little girl, "I'm sorry that things happened to us to make us believe we weren't good enough." I told her it wasn't her fault to believe things about us that were not true because we were young and kids always think everything is their fault, even when people are mean to them. I told her that she did the best job she could have possibly done for us at the time. I assured her I knew better now because God told me so. She smiled at me as I watched her heart heal. Then she ran off with a full heart to play with a group of kids, knowing she was good enough.

Looking back I can see my actions during the majority of my life, and cancer treatment, through the eyes of my seven-year-old self. Only trying to protect myself from more pain, not knowing any other way. I now look at myself with empathy for living like that and realize that, even though misguided, it was still heroic. I was willing to make the effort every day to lift my *more than* shield. I never gave up and always continued to move forward in this world with a smile on my face and determination in my heart, giving it my best effort to not be *less than.* That effort took a lot of strength too. Now I know it required too much human strength for a seven-year-old girl or a forty-eight-year-old woman. I am glad I found God and no longer need to wear myself out listening to my false beliefs.

I think everyone comes up with the best strategy available when they are younger based on their genetics, experiences, and surroundings—whether they are withdrawing, deflecting, or shielding themselves from their *less than* minds. In order to stop hurting ourselves and others everyone's journey needs a force greater than humanness to save them from their mind's judgment of weakness. That is where God shows up in our stories— to help us change our mind's so we can change our lives.

If you had met me, prior to cancer, I would never have told you that I ever felt *less than* about anything. Well, sometimes my weight, but other than that I would have told you that my life's résumé showed that I was not only good enough but that I had a better batting average than a lot of people. I was never even aware of why I worked so hard at everything and became upset when I felt rejected or disrespected. I never conceived that my behavior was a result of a subconscious belief that I needed to stop people from rejecting me. I just thought that was my personality. I didn't know it was done in self-defense against my mind—until I got cancer. Now I can see the deceptive game I played with myself. I went through life claiming victories beneath the labels of my house, my kids, my job, or whatever success I could use to shield myself from my subconscious feelings of inadequacy and belief that I would again be rejected because I was *less than* others.

PART 6

The Rise

Those closest to death know each other in divine ways that are incomprehensible to others. There is an unspoken knowing of each other. Even though I went to a hospital that treated people with every type of cancer under the sun, I would always somehow know who had breast cancer. They would recognize me too. I decided that when you are that sick, your angels and their angels whisper to each other to find out what you need. My sisters and I were somehow able to overhear their conversations, allowing us to know the Truth of each other without saying a word. It still takes my breath away thinking about all the times that I was exactly where I needed to be to meet one of my sisters and give one of them what they needed at the right moment, or receive from them exactly what I needed at that moment. Our angels put us where we needed to be, trying to save our lives.

Evelyn. I still say her name often to myself. Her name is blessed to me now. I will always remember what she looks like, yet sometimes her image in my mind is softened, like in a dream. I had first noticed her as I turned around, hoping to make the six or so steps to one of two available chairs behind me. I was trying to make this necessary transition since leaning on the counter of the hospital's sign-in desk for support was no longer, physically, a practical option. My mom continued to check me in for my appointments as I clumsily landed in the safety of the chair to assume my familiar hunched position, head down, back curved.

I was yet again sitting in the bustling atrium lobby of the cancer hospital. It was 6:30 in the morning. After arriving in Chicago less than ten hours before with the newly ripe orange in my breast and having cried most of the night, I had only managed to get a couple of hours' sleep. If you could have seen my hidden heart, you would have known that I was emotionally and physically drained. The payoff for that was that *fear* barely had enough oxygen to smolder. The other side of that meant that there wasn't nearly enough oxygen for me to breathe.

Unable to find enough air in my bosom, I lifted my head, searching for breath outside of me. I was again scanning my environment to see if anything was different. This time it was. As I lifted my head, I again caught a glance of this beautiful, petite, olive-skinned woman in her early sixties dressed in a white, soft-cotton T-shirt, ankle-length, flowing white skirt, and tan sandals standing across the room. I thought she looked out of place because she had long, silky black hair with gentle curls, and wore beautiful, natural-looking makeup, including soft pink lipstick. You do not see too many people put together that nicely at the cancer hospital, especially at that time of the morning. As I was taking in the sight of her, she turned her head, and with her dark brown eyes looked right into my heart. I could not take my eyes off her. She intuitively moved toward me, and I somehow knew that she was supposed to come to me. She effortlessly glided into the chair next to me without a word being exchanged between us. She leaned over and cupped her hand over mine. She said, "I'm Evelyn. I have breast cancer, stage four," and then nonchalantly, "but that's just a number." I said, "I'm Carol. I have breast cancer too, and my tumor just grew back." I instinctively offered her my other hand, like a small child reaching for its mother's safety. She immediately accepted my offering and started praying for me.

For some reason, it was understood between us that she would do that. I was still new and awkward when praying to God, making her ease with God mystifying to me. When I heard her words, I couldn't believe that she was praying for the same things that I had talked about with God the night before. As she continued speaking with God, her words were then directed to me. Evelyn's words from God gave me answers to the questions I was asking God the night before and assurances about what was going to happen to me. My simple prayers always lacked any sort of stamina. She prayed for almost five minutes. I couldn't even take in all the words at that moment; I was too overwhelmed by her presence. As I drifted among her words, I remember feeling honored and humbled that she was praying to God just for me. I somehow knew she was sent to me, just for me, from God. She was the miracle I asked God for. Evelyn told me, "Do not worry. You're going to be fine. Everything is going to be okay." I knew her words were from God and were not platitudes; lifting away from my shoulders the fear of the tumor's reappearance. The heaviness that had me searching for breath floated up to the top of the atrium, and my body became uplifted and light. I felt like a hundred-pound weight had been taken from me. Apparently Evelyn was to leave on a shuttle to go to the airport; the driver and other passengers were waiting for her as she was praying. After reentering the world at the close of her prayer, I looked up and saw that everyone was silent and reverent as they witnessed our interaction. Everyone was captivated watching my beautiful angel Evelyn answering my prayer for a miracle from God.

At 6:40 a.m., I sat peacefully in the hospital atrium, the only space in the hospital where sunlight managed to shine on everyone. I was registered for a day of doctors, blood tests, and scans, to see what my fate would be. However, I already knew that I would be okay. Evelyn had given me a heads-up from God. I easily rose, even with the orange lodged in my right breast, and walked to the elevator. As I waited for the doors to open, I realized that I was standing right where the haunting vision from my first visit occurred. I had found myself in the exact same spot where I first saw the woman in the blue and white scarf bent over in her wheelchair. As I stood there, now in the shoes of a woman who herself had sat hunched over in a wheelchair, I lifted my head a bit and fully straightened my back. As I did so I humbly acknowledged my miracle, believing that everything was going to be okay. I didn't know how to make it okay. I just knew it *would* be.

Evelyn was the turning point for me. I could no longer shake off the coincidences of Truth. I now absolutely knew that my encounters with the divine were not happening willy-nilly. What I did not know at the time was that awakening and staying awake long enough to fully awaken were two different things.

The Three Amigos. The one cancer god, the oncologist who had told me to do chemo before surgery out of fear the cancer had spread, was now telling me to do the surgery over more chemo, out of fear the cancer had spread. The other cancer god, who had said that tumors did not grow back in a few weeks and could only quote the FDA guidelines like a robot, did not have an explanation or protocol or for this, so she also wanted me to do surgery. The third cancer god felt that, since I had become so sick from doing chemo, delaying doing more chemo on the right schedule, I had what he called "incomplete" treatment, and I should do more chemo.

Later that day, after the miracle of Evelyn, I was in a gown in an examination room. My least favorite cancer god, the oncologist that refused to let me do surgery after my second chemo, walked into the examining room and audibly gasped when she saw the orange in my breast. When your oncologist now cannot breathe right either, you know that you were right all along about the lack of air in this place. When she found enough breath to speak, she now stood inside of my fear-based nightmare and exclaimed in astonishment and disbelief, "I have never seen such a thing!" She immediately said that I needed a mammogram and PET scan and quickly rushed out of the room with no other words of reassurance for me. Her eyes only left a shock wave of fear and unknowing about what was happening to me. She again shut the door on me. My mom and I immediately looked at each other.

We were now more stunned from her reaction than from the orange sitting in my breast.

After the mammogram, it was determined that the inside of the orange only contained my previous tumor. It had regrown and was now 75 percent of its original size. The remainder of the orange mass was my body's tissue trying to encapsulate and protect me from the cancer. I opted not to have the PET scan. I chose to believe Evelyn: that the cancer had not spread anywhere else.

When you are overly drugged and in so deep, you feel that everything is pretty much lost. You don't understand that cancer treatment plays a cruel game. Players are surrounded by lights and noises, creating an atmosphere that makes them feel drunk, all to masquerade the dishonesty just like in Vegas. The calculated chaos stops you from realizing that the house usually wins. This allows you to reason that when you are down to your final dollar you might as well place everything you have left on the roulette wheel, all on red, instead of holding on to the last bit of your life and saying 'enough'. You want to believe that the joke has not been on you, that this time the gambler will beat the odds and hit the jackpot.

I acted like the abused kids I had watched on television, who screamed for the parent who just beat them as the authorities were taking the child away. Even with all their bruises, their connection with that parent was the only safety they knew, not knowing life could be any other way.

Although Evelyn had told me I was going to be okay, she had not told me *how* to be okay. I had no idea what to do to fix myself. I felt that the only thing to hold on to was chemo because that is all I had known. That is what I was made to believe would heal me. I thought all my days on the couch, in the hospital, and all the damage to my body from the chemo had just gone up in flames. All of it was for nothing. How could I have paid such a high price and told myself that the end—saving my life—justified the means of destroying my body? I needed to rebuild my web… my chemo web. I felt I was "pot committed" as they say in poker. I still wanted certainty. I wanted to see the tumor go away again, thinking that would make me feel safe again. I decided that I wanted to do a fifth round of A/C (Adriamycin and Cytoxan) chemo since it had worked so well initially. For some reason I only remembered how it kicked the tumor's butt and forgot the part about it kicking mine. The nurses call A/C the Red Devil; its dark maroon hue looks like evil, and as one of the most powerful chemo regimens it has many devastating side effects including severe heart damage. The Devil and I were split at this point. I won the first two rounds and he won the last two. I wanted to believe I was due to win this round.

The two oncologists from the cut-it-out camp would not administer the Devil, saying that the probability of heart damage was too high after four rounds. The more-chemo guy was up for more, not concerned about my heart. At that point, I didn't trust anyone. They could not even agree with each other, and believing in their collective wisdom had left me with an orange-sized lump in my breast. Fear tells you to keep moving forward, even harder. Doing more of the same and expecting different results is how it is done in the world of fear.

The way out of your mind and into your faith is when you can accept and see yourself as God sees you. The Christian faith offers Jesus' gift of taking judgment from the world, including your mean mind, and offering blanket forgiveness to everyone, including yourself. Know that when you are upset with a person or circumstance you are sitting outside of your Truth. You are no longer in the safe place of love. When your life is failing, love is gone and fear rules.

"He that loves his brother abides in the light, and there is no occasion of stumbling in him. But he that hates his brother is in darkness, and walks in darkness, and knows not where he goes, because that darkness has blinded his eyes." John 2:10-11

By now I had got the message loud and clear; I had cancer. Even though I did not want to remember much of the past four months, I knew I did not sign a release form for a lobotomy. Why did they strip me of all my dignity because I got cancer? Why was I no longer me: a wife, mother, businesswoman, daughter, friend, or sister, but *just* a *less than* cancer patient? Who decided that when you get cancer you have to give up your *person card*? People who have heart attacks don't have to do that. The truth is they do not even ask you to give it up. Without care or thought they frisk you, taking any remaining possessions and remnants of your life. The familiar parts of you are then put in a sanitized clear bag and placed on a high shelf in full view, but just out of reach. All you are is your cancer.

I was talked at and talked about, scared to death with inaccurate facts and assessments, and monotone explanations that I knew had been said on autoplay. The standard protocol is scheduled to keep your head spinning. You are looking for any place to be still and be *you*. But the cancer parade is in full swing and you need to march in lockstep with the other sheep for the shearing, and maybe the slaughter. You are prodded to follow the herd because you are branded and your destiny has been pre-ordained by the cancer gods; the oncologists. You know questions are discouraged and obedience is demanded because you don't know what they know about cancer. See; they know the odds and the statistics are stacked against you and they are willing to sacrifice your life on the off chance that they might save it. If you dare speak up, their response is, "That's rare; this symptom and that symptom don't happen much. I've never seen that before." They also know that as their chemo drugs continue to flow through your mind and body, your objections will be silenced. Even though you do not believe in them, you now believe in yourself less. It's not their medicine; it's you. Your blood pressure's high, your sugar's high, your kidneys are struggling, your liver enzymes are high, and you're anemic. It is not us and the chemicals we call medicine that we put in you. It's your body, your lousy cancer body having problems. It took me a while to catch on, but after three stays in the hospital, I began to think, *Gee if I am the weak link here, why is there a whole floor of cancer patients in this hospital?*

After the MRSA, I became incensed at the whole process back to day one, especially at the oncologist who would not let me have surgery when I begged for it. I was irate. My mom told me to let it go, and I tried, but could not do it completely. I carried the anger and hatred of what was done to me around until the tumor came back. After feeling betrayed to the point of almost losing my life, I watched death grow back. That's when I sarcastically said, "The only way to prove I'm right about the medical profession, the FDA, the drug companies, the insurance companies, and everyone else involved in this debacle they call medicine, is to die." I lost my breath when I said those words.

I knew at that point, when I said those words about having to die to prove I was right, that I would have to forgive everything about what medicine had done to me under the guise of doing it for me, or I was going to die. I had to forgive the doctor who would not let me have the surgery when I pleaded with her for it. I had to let every bit of the resentment and betrayal I felt from her actions and other doctors go, or I would die. It was really that simple. *That knowing* was black and white. Whatever choice I made, I knew what the outcome would be. I chose life. My life was more important than proving how they broke their oath to "first do no harm." My life was more important than being right about the mistakes they made and dying to prove how wrong they were. When you understand life in those terms, you see how ridiculous it is not to forgive anything, and why you need to forgive everything, including yourself.

Back then, trying to forgive felt unnatural, but I knew I had to do it. I did not have time for a therapist, so I decided to ask God to help me forgive. I had to make peace with it all now, and I only knew one place that I had ever found peace was with God. I had to hand it over to God to hold for me because I could not possess that anger for one more deadly second. I had people tell me, "Let go and let God," and, "Give it up to God." I had no idea how to do this, but with no other viable plan available, I tried. I found out that you cannot just wish anger away as I had tried to do when my Mom told me to let it go. I also couldn't do it by snapping my impatient fingers and demanding it to leave. I had to be in my heart, not my head, before I could release it. I had to open my heart and sit in the earnest peace of my Truth when I asked God to take it, and He did. I again found my way to my Truth to do this because I wanted to live. I let it all go because I needed love to heal my heart, and the resentment from not forgiving was stopping that from happening.

This is how I learned that Truth is black and white. There is no gray. You are either in your Truth or not. Now, whenever I think that a situation is gray, I peacefully sit within the brightly lit holy space of Truth and can easily see the shadow cast by the lie. I know that I cannot have my heart in Truth if I am still listening to my mind in the lie. I have to be all in. Until anything is wholly given up to God, all of it will remain as a barrier to God. The Truth is never a win-or-lose proposition. It is always a win. Sometimes it is a human struggle to get there, but the divine awaits you. I then knew that if I wanted to choose life, I had to always commit to forgiveness.

Many people then and now have told me I have every right to be angry about what happened to me during my treatment. That is true; it is my right. I have the choice to feel however I want to feel about anything. That's why I chose to let it go and forgive because my right to be angry contradicted my decision to live and heal my heart. You cannot be angry and find the necessary love and peace that will heal your heart. It did not matter how right I thought I was and how wrong I believed they were. My only choice, in order to live, was to release my anger. I chose to forgive everyone and live in peace; not for them but for me. Their initial blows had been life-threatening enough. I was not going to hold on to their actions and put my life on the line every day forward, continuing to do the same thing to myself. My bottom-line choice for life was to not give my heart one more second of their pain. I needed my heart to heal in order to live, and I needed peace for that to happen.

Today, when I look back, I honestly believe every one of my doctors was doing the best they knew how. Sure, it could have been better, but I don't think anyone was trying to kill me. They too are human beings with imperfect minds and actions. I was requiring them to perform the work of God. I now take responsibility for not understanding that the business of being a doctor of medicine is confined to a narrow approach of healing possibilities. It does not reach far beyond what is allowed by government regulations, insurance company reimbursements, and what drugs the hospital wants to sell to patients from the pharmaceutical companies. I gave these practitioners of medicine much more authority and responsibility for healing me than I should have. Some drugs may have their place in healing, but they are not the sole answer to curing humans who are more than just a body. When the human mind interacts and causes the human body to malfunction, it must also be healed. I needed to take responsibility for rebalancing what medicine had to offer with what my mind needed: God. Finding God gave me enough peace to open myself up to the greatest possibility of healing.

After I realized that I ran my world trying to protect myself from my *less than* mind, I realized everyone does this to some degree one way or another. This is why we must forgive everyone for everything, including ourselves.

My *less than* mind always had me working overtime to earn the approval of my bosses and customers. Knowing they appreciated my zealousness to deliver plus-one service eased my mind's pronouncements. What I did not realize at the time was that my need for acceptance caused me to sometimes place over-zealous requirements on my co-workers. I was trying to be *more than,* to protect myself from my mind. In turn, I created stress for others. I didn't do it to be hurtful; I was doing the best I knew how at that time.

Now, when anyone behaves badly toward me or someone else, I know they are running their world as I did and sometimes still do: trying to protect themselves from their *less than* pronouncements in their mind. When people try to protect themselves by acting as an assailant trying to puff themselves up, put me down, steal, lie, control, judge, or otherwise hurt me, it stems from their mind's pain. I can now step back after the initial shock, hurt, or anger I experience from their actions, and know that they are doing the best they can trying to defend themselves from their *less than* minds.

This does not mean I exempt their behavior from rules, regulations, and laws necessary to address and provide consequences for their actions. But I also try my best to not throw my hurt from their actions back into their pile of pain, by knowing that it must already be at a tipping point for them to act that way. In addition, I also try to arrange my life from that point forward, to not give them the same opportunity to hurt me or my loved ones again. However, the most important thing I do is to understand that their bad behavior is about them, not me. I do not take it personally, as a reflection of my *less than* thinking, as I did in the past. I keep *their* pain where it belongs: with *their* mind's *less than* thinking that they have acted upon. I refuse to hold any resentment or hurt resulting from *their* behavior, because that is *their* pain and not mine to hold. I simply forgive their *less than* mind's actions so my *less than* mind will not grab hold of it and make it my pain. I let it go and wholeheartedly move on with my peaceful life.

Cancer treatment did not give me courage. I had somehow, in the unrelenting, pelting rain of horror, learned that my fear lay only in what I had known, not what I didn't. To survive, I had to know of things I could not explain. When courage was not enough and I was not enough, I found a morsel of belief and became more than enough the moment I handed over everything that I had to God.

"And I will bring the blind by a way that they knew not; I will lead them in paths that they have not known: I will make darkness light before them, and crooked things straight. These things will I do unto them, and not forsake them." Isaiah 42:16

In the beginning, before I noticed the divine crumbs of destiny, I followed the trail of fear. It was familiar to me. The same sights, sounds, and thoughts I had always followed were now just more amplified by the cancer. I knew how to navigate these trails and believed I could use what I had learned of them to fight cancer. I moved and thought as fast as I could, trying to outrun cancer with my swift and sure footing that had brought me all my previously believed victories. The problem that someone on this trail faces is that all the noise stops you from thinking clearly. You pay attention to the racket and it drowns out your real voice. You choose your blinders so you can run faster and not become distracted from the race. I was so enchanted by the trail that it never occurred to me that it was the very path that led me to cancer.

So there I was, running as fast I could, almost out of breath, yet further in the wrong direction. I believed in the magic potion of chemotherapy the trail billboards advertised. I was convinced that something outside of me would save me. The signage on this trail was deceptive: nice house, law degree, great vacations, and six-figure salary this way.

My progression in the wrong direction was abruptly halted by one of the most deadly infections today: MRSA. When I got kicked in the butt by MRSA and was unable to move, the doctors then dragged me further down the dead-end trail. At that point, unable to lift my head up off the rock-hard path, I became disorientated. I had lost my balance and could no longer navigate the trail. I had to crawl off of it on my hands and knees in the middle of the dark night, knowing it was leading me to my death. I did not even know if there was any other way. All I knew was there was no point in going any farther that way. I lay there disconnected, lost without hope. I couldn't even cry. In order to cry you have to think something could be different. I did not know there was any other way of being in the world I had created. When there was nothing to cry out to and I had no strength left to form tears anyway, I sat there numb and hopeless until I decided to look for a new way.

At first I didn't even know if there was another path, but I knew that not looking meant I was at this trail's end and it was time to die. As I slowly sat up, I began to sense something was different. I was beginning to see my way outside of the old way and began to see my surroundings in a different light. Still trying to navigate this decision with limited skills, I somehow understood that I needed to walk slowly and pay attention in order to ensure that, even if I stumbled, I wouldn't fall unconscious, allowing me to rise again and continue on. It was then, when I was too tired to move forward or had my head down, that I would find a divine crumb from God that would nourish me a bit. I began to notice the divine morsels more and more. Then I began seeking them out. The sustenance was not laid evenly but rather it meandered through some pretty rocky terrain. At the end of the trail, I found perfection in its path. The nourishment fed my body, healed my heart, and helped me build my bridge to God.

The old me would have preferred having God scoop me up and place me back on my misguided path in an unchanged direction so I could get on with my old life. Had that been done, I would not have found my way back to whom I really was, not the me who got cancer but the me of God. Many people do not. I feel honored that I was allowed to run, stumble, fall, lie, sit, claw, crawl, rest, stand, and walk to God… then, most importantly, hold the hand of God. My journey included a series of fires that sometimes burned me, sometimes warmed me, and sometimes left a few scars. After the physical fire always came the internal storm. Pounding thunder, piercing lightning, and heavy rain that scared me, required great surrender, and at the same time cleansed me. In the forest that could be desolate and sometimes treacherous, I also found bountiful offerings and refuge from the fervor and the tears. Although it took me awhile to understand the nuances of my nature, I began to recognize the transformative balance of form and light, and my ability to experience pain and restoration from the very same composition of the flames and downpours. I learned to navigate the obstacles of my mind and listen for the voice of God. Every step I took and every breath I received made me more aware of a place I had not yet remembered. I am honored to be with God to walk and hold His hand every day with the peace He brings me in my heart.

If you ever wonder what happens in the chasm, know that as you fall you lose parts of you that you thought knew better, leaving the parts of you that you don't remember to fend for you.

When you are too sick to sit up, you have to hunch over. When you cannot stand up and walk without leaning on another person—and even that taxes all of your will and swipes your last bit of energy. When everything aches, you're nauseated, and you know that your body is barely keeping up with the fight. When you are conscious yet cannot form thoughts on a regular basis, and if words do come, you can barely find the energy to whisper them. When all you can do is watch not partake. When you have to quietly stare and stare and stare at what you are now an outsider to, day after day, week after week, month after month. This is *when* your pain marinates with your separateness uncontrollably taking hold of you, putting you in a free fall down the chasm of isolation. This is *when* you become lost inside of a place that is deep and hidden, a place that is so far away from life *here*, so far down from consciousness, that you become unreachable.

For someone who was always used to winning, who knew how to play the player and play the game, this was inconceivable. I was smart and could think outside of the box. My words made things happen at work and at home. I also had enormous physical strength. I had been an athlete and was tall and always strong both mentally and physically. I was living my heroic illusion until I woke up in my *less than* nightmare.

The force of the descent no longer allowed me to hold the broken parts of me together, causing the sharpest and shiniest pieces of me to fall off into the dark gorge and shatter. By the time I realized that this was happening those coveted parts of me were already gone. All that remained was an uncomfortable twinge as I tried to search my thoughts for a remembrance of them. I became disorientated and void in my brokenness. Everything I knew and valued had vanished from my world.

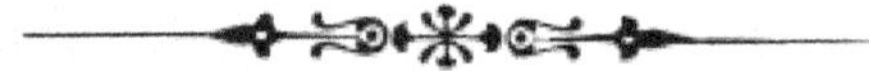

"And He is before all things, and by Him all things are held together."
Colossians 1:17

In less than two months, I had been in the hospital three times, had one more round of chemo, lost thirty pounds, and had my tumor grow back. It all happened so quickly. I forfeited pieces of me at such a fast clip that I desperately tried to hold on to whatever was left. As I tried to clutch onto my disappearing world, I only pushed myself further into the nothingness. I thought that I had lost everything of anything that made me matter. As I was tumbling through the chasm so hard and too fast, I traveled upside down or sideways for the greater part of the fall. This meant everything appeared to me in jumbled snapshots with no logical connection. As I was breaking apart, I could not grasp how to even hold on to what was left, let alone put anything back together.

I had quietly broken when I was in the hospital for the first time and the surgical resident made me beg for my life. In my attempt to save my life, I conceded what was left of anything that I thought made me matter. I handed it over to the medical student in my desperate negotiations for one more day of care. That is when the propped-up pieces of me shattered and scattered out of my grip. I spoke this out loud for the first time a little over a month later at my prep appointment for my fifth round of potentially heart-stopping chemo from the Red Devil.

At lunchtime, I went to a healthy-cooking class at the more-chemo doctor's clinic. I found a seat among the other cancer patients and their caregivers. As I quietly sat there, I realized that I was unable to participate as I had done before in these demonstrations. I felt that I had gone to the other side of somewhere. All the days on my couch and in my hospital bed, when my body could not move I had felt this way, but to again be displaced like this after my strength had returned was shocking. I could again walk and talk, yet, to my disbelief, I suddenly and fully experienced that the same disconnection from *Here* I suffered during all those long days of staring and staring. I now knew it was actually real. I was neither *Here* with my mind nor *Over There* with God. It was the first time I became consciously aware of the pit in which I sat. I did not have a label for it at the time and became anxious and confused, not knowing where I was or where I belonged—but very aware that it was not at this cooking seminar.

The leader of the demonstration then asked me a simple question: "How are you doing?" Even though it was just a token gesture, I frightfully exclaimed without thinking, "I'm broken." My mind started reeling as I thought, *Wait… what… WHAT? Me—broken? Why would I say that? I bend; I don't break… just like the song. What part of my chemoed brain came up with the word broken?* But once I'd said it, I could not take it back and pretend it wasn't true. Broken is broken, and saying it ain't so doesn't fix it. I had broken. I was broken. It's lonely to know you are broken. It's even lonelier when you see in other people's eyes and hear in their voices that they know you are broken too.

To fix broken, you must have most of the pieces to assemble what once was. I did not. I had to nurture and grow what were once subtle parts of me to fill in the big holes of what had to be broken and lost to save my life while embracing God's love to smooth out the rough edges.

A divine crumb of truth revealed as a passing random thought lures in the tide. Waves continually lap against me as I stand with my back toward the ocean. Suddenly the next wave that rolls in is a direct hit against my body with an unseen undercurrent. Water bursts in all directions beneath me, throwing my shocked framework forward to my knees. Once on my knees I am taken under, twisting so violently that I hold my breath, only to choke on it as I scramble to find my way back to the surface. And when the ocean again allows me to rise, I am now facing the mystical horizon through the vastness of the water not yet understanding that I was now facing Over There.

When I was sick, I stared and stared and stared out at the world going on around me. I found myself exiled behind a one-way mirrored window that I could look out of but no one could look in. Knowing me, I probably put the mirror on it so no one would have to see that I was gone. I was lonely and desperately wanted to get back *Here*, get back through that reflecting closed window to where my world was going on without me. However, I did not have the physical strength to break through.

I had no choice but to let it go, continuing to stare and stare. As a prisoner, I dreamed of my escape to come, when my physical strength returned to rescue me. At the healthy-lunch event that day, my physical strength had returned. It was then I became aware that it was not just my body but my *mind* that had stumbled into brokenness. Now I knew my isolation was more than in my physical being. My mind now held me prisoner to that which my body did not. I was devastated when my mind shut the blind on my window so I could no longer even watch what my life used to be *Here.* I could not articulate it then, but I somehow intuitively knew that if I crossed the pane to my old life, I would die.

At that moment, I felt like the guy on *Planet of the Apes* who spent the whole movie trying to get back to the United States so he could escape the nightmare of where his spaceship had landed. When he finally made it back to his spacecraft, he realized it was sitting outside of the Lincoln Memorial in Washington, D.C. There was no way out. Where he didn't want to be was exactly where he wanted to go. When where you don't want to be and where you want to be are the same place, you need to change your mind about one of them. The limbo of the chasm is where you sit until you make a new choice.

I had to find a way to make what was unfamiliar comfortable, and accept that where I thought I wanted to be, *here*, was somewhere I could not live as I had before. I felt like an outsider in my own inner life. I was going to have to learn to befriend my new world *here* or resist it and die. To find my way out of my exile, I needed to build a bridge back to God first. Until then I would remain a prisoner in the nowhereness of my *less than* chasm.

Once I began to pay attention, I started to notice everything my new world offered. I found that sometimes I would find my way outside of the feeling of being nowhere, but only when I experienced things that brought me love or joy; like my kids… especially my kids.

But not if they were fighting. When they were fighting, I drifted away back into the discomfort of the chasm. As time passed, I began to notice that the times I felt free to reenter my new world, which was my old world, I had to have love or joy in my heart to do so. As quickly as love or joy would allow me to enter, negativity would send me right back to the depths.

That was when I began to start all over, to recast myself. I had to adapt myself to what is not what was and accept that everything had changed. I had to assimilate with the monkeys of my mind. I needed to create a crossing between my human mind and God's love. To find happiness in my new version of my old world, I had to find my way beyond my former thoughts of what and how it should look and be. I began to understand I could only be *Here* with love or joy from *Over There*, with God. Anything that caused pain or distress happened now in the old world *less than* thinking and wanting what I believed it had been, without God. As I learned to live in this new place, I began to remember and recognize the unfamiliar as familiar and recognize precious parts of me that were lost in my old world thinking. So now, the not-much-of-anything, nothing familiar, nothing interesting, and always painful, were the last forty-plus years of my life when I was not with God. Looking back and recounting my best memories of those years, they were always of times where love or joy was present.

I remember reading *Walden* by Henry David Thoreau when I was in college. I never forgot his words that "the mass of men lead lives of quiet desperation." I always thought that would be a sad way to go through life. I never saw myself though that lens or consciously felt the despair I thought he was talking about. But the truth is I secretly and subconsciously covered up my mind's anguish so well I couldn't even acknowledge my pain and desperation. It turns out I *was* one of the masses he was talking about, when I lived my life without God.

Unmerited favor is described in the Bible through Jesus' offering of forgiveness and eternal life as a free gift that cannot be fought for or earned. Some take the high road; some take the low road. I always took the toll road, not knowing that someone else's love had already paid.

I was back home after completing my fifth attempt with the Red Devil. This treatment of A/C was only seventy-five percent of the standard dosing to reduce my potential heart attack by twenty-five percent I guess. Due to the smaller dosage, I was feeling okay—not great, but my face was not stuck to the couch. I knew that even if this worked and I won this round with cancer, I still had a really high chance of it coming back. I found this out when, without my asking, one of the cancer gods pronounced to me that my reoccurrence odds, since the tumor grew back, now greatly exceeded the sixty percent ceiling the Internet had previously calculated.

As I was sitting on the couch in my living room and thinking about my life after my treatments were over, I pictured myself on vacation with my kids, playing on a beach, and then, *bam!...* My mind was filled with fear about the statistics, percentages, and stories I'd heard about cancer returning. I felt fear would always be hanging in the air around me, overpowering any joy or fun. I didn't know how anyone could ever have an enjoyable life after cancer. How would I ever spend one day in peace without the thought, *I hope it doesn't come back?* It felt like winning was too conditional, too tenuous, and too scary. It made me feel like my best days were behind me. Nothing would ever be carefree again. Even if I had been living in an illusion of my web of security, it sure was more comfortable than my new reality of Russian roulette. I pictured myself wasting whatever was left of my life by wishing away my precious days until enough had passed to give me a safe enough distance away from the dark cancer cloud. I would have to check off today, tomorrow, and the next day, until I hit the magic number that dropped my risk of reoccurrence percentage low enough to keep my fear at a tolerable level. Of course knowing that the overwhelming odds were that I would not make it to the other side of the count down.

I then stood up after bantering these thoughts in my mind and began walking from the living room through the dining room toward our open galley kitchen. I began contemplating how and when the next shoe was going to drop. When I lifted my head out of my thoughts, I glanced outside through the bay window at the far end of the kitchen. I noticed it was a beautiful sunny July day. Then a life changing thought arose. I thought, *I don't have to get cancer back anymore and then beat it.* I was not paying attention to my thoughts at that point and assumed that I had misunderstood what I had just said to myself.

Confused, I stopped walking and just stood there. That pause allowed the thought to resurface again: *I don't have to get cancer back anymore and then beat it.* Then more came: *That would be a complete waste of time. I've done that trick with everything my entire life. The dark horse winning is now a tired out, boring game that I have played my whole life. I don't have to do this the hard way like everything else. I don't have to get cancer back and then win.* I then started smiling and thinking, *Wow—I don't have to get cancer back, fight it, and then win? I don't have to get it back? Wait… what… WHAT?* Then a laugh choked out a noise of escaping trapped air from my mouth. This expelling of the lie I had been holding most of my life allowed me to inhale the fresh air that had been elusive to me for the past five months… and the past forty-plus years.

This was the first time I ever remember having a thought like that, a consideration that I didn't have to do something the hard way. My life's story to that point had always revolved around overcoming adversity. Everything that I had won, earned, or achieved I did it the hard way. I hated watching football games where one team was down by fourteen or more points at halftime. I always knew how they felt. They not only had to score as much as the other team in the second half but then score two more touchdowns and a field goal to win. It's not fun when you always have to play from behind, but that's how I had run my world. I always believed that I had to do twice as much as everyone to win, and that is how it always went for me. The good news is, I had a pretty good track record of coming back and winning. The bad news is it made life so flipping hard.

Of course, I did not figure out that I didn't have to do it the hard way until *after* my tumor grew back. So there it was: the realization that I didn't have to struggle and strive to come from behind with an extra rock on my back every time, holding my shield of my *more thans* and fighting my way up the mountain all day every day, against the *less thans* in my mind. Always trying to try to catch up with everyone else, then somehow finding the energy to not only make it the rest of the way, but beat them to the finish. On an ordinary sunny day, I had a single thought that changed my life. On that day, the rocks that I had carried on my back one by one, day by day, to the top of a steep mountain that built my *more than* tower that imprisoned me imploded!

The Truth about mirrors. ***Mirrors reflect back how your mind sees you. God sees something different from behind your reflection. As you stand in front of the mirror and extend your arm to punch what you see as yourself, you realize that you would never win a fight with the image you see in the mirror. Only your human body can be physically hurt. The mind's image in the mirror is untouchable no matter how hard you strike. If you want to know who you really are, then you have to step inside the mirror behind the mind's picture of you. You will then be standing as an untouchable wholeness that cannot be hurt by your mind's pretense and will be able to look out at your human self. From this angle, you will be humbled by what you see. Why? Because from inside the mirror, you know that your mind's false perception stops at its bent image of you. From behind the mind's shining false view nothing can harm you and you are safe to know the Truth about yourself. You will look at yourself from a place of peace and stillness. You will see yourself with compassion and love. You will know yourself as God does. You will only see perfection. There are no blemishes from***

inside the mirror looking out. Only when you are outside the mirror looking through your mind's eyes can you perceive imperfection.

When flying from Jamestown, North Dakota to Chicago O'Hare Airport, I always had a layover in Minneapolis. I would fly in on small planes from Jamestown to Minneapolis. These planes were not large enough to use a jet bridge, so I would exit down the stairs from the aircraft onto the runway and walk about a hundred yards to the terminal. Once inside the building, I was too physically weak to walk the great distance to the elevator, making the stairs my best option. I would have to find the strength to make my way up two flights of stairs to the terminal to catch my next flight. What took even greater effort was pushing down my humiliation and uncomfortably asking an airline employee for help to carry my roller bag up the stairs.

I would then grasp on to the handrail, desperately wishing for the energy to make it up the stairs as fast as I could. Each step was a futile attempt to outpace my shame as the airline employee now waited at the top of the stairs with my bag. I wanted to explain my situation once I made it to the top of the stairs, but was always too tired and too embarrassed so I just thanked them and apologized too much for being such an inconvenience. I usually had this conversation with my head down because I was struggling to catch my breath. As soon as I was able to lift my head I would eye the closest chair.

I would then begin my walk of shame toward that crucial resting spot. As I slowly moved toward my seat, I felt my body flinch as I received the pity in the air from other travelers' stares of confusion and questioning about the sad condition of a woman my age. I would then drop my head, unable to make eye contact with the world. I had to let go of its grip. I had to pretend that I was not there so everyone's looks would stop hurting me. I would then fall into the first available chair, exhausted. I would sit there hunched over, not only to catch my breath but simply because I did not have the physical strength to sit up. I would stare and stare at the blue carpet under my feet, unsuccessfully keeping my tears from falling on it as I tried to focus my thoughts on finding the energy and will to get to my next gate. I was holding on as tight as I could and fearing that I could not do it much longer. When I ran out of time to rest, I would then close my eyes and force myself to stand up. Once I steadied myself, I would try to lift my legs and push them clumsily in front of me like a child learning how to walk, attempting to move forward and make it to my next gate… for my connecting fight to the cancer hospital.

As I was going for my later chemos, I started having a vision of myself doing this. Not when I was dreaming, or even when my eyes were closed—I could easily see the vision whenever I was sitting quietly and staring off. The vision started out simply: I would watch myself from the vantage point of someone standing several feet behind me as I was walking up the ramp to go to my connecting gate. I would feel this great love and compassion for myself as I stood there watching myself. Once I had this vision, it would surface a couple of times a week in my thoughts. The vision continued to grow the more I opened up to it.

Here is the entire vision, narrated by my female voice of God:

"I stand behind her in the airport terminal. Watching her hunched over and struggling to put one foot in front of the other, walking up the long inclined hallway to her connecting gate. Her clothes are baggy, and I know that she doesn't know how crooked the fake blonde hair is under that red baseball cap. Her face is a pale yellow, swollen ball from the drugs. Her brown eyes are sunk in and sad… deeply sad. She needs more than she can even know. The only thing she can think about now is successfully putting together some sort of rhythm to exchange her back foot with the front foot in order to move forward."

"I watch her from behind as a mother does when her child starts to walk. I want to be there to catch her if she falls. I offer all of myself to give her enough love to carry her steps forward. I love her and want to take care of her. I will do anything I can for her. She is special and she's mine. I ache and silently cry, watching her suffering. My heart weeps for her, but I know something she doesn't: she will not only make it to her gate, but she will beat cancer. I quietly whisper this to her as she is losing her breath and slowing her pace. She hears me and wants to believe it, but she just does not know where my voice is coming from. At least, thinking it might be true, she can continue forward. I know she is so loving and determined."

I am not sure where this vision came from. Some people have told me the woman's voice is my angel. But it does not matter who she is; she is of God and she loves me. This vision allowed me to start seeing myself differently. Not as someone who was judged and *less than,* but as someone who was wholly loved and being watched, guided and cared for from a place I did not know existed. I now, for the first time, felt complete unconditional love and utter compassion for myself, the same way I would have if I were watching my own child suffering. I now saw myself as someone who didn't need to earn every scrap of love and acceptance that was given. When I felt I was at my most unworthy, unable to do anything for anyone to earn acceptance, I somehow was shown that I was good enough to receive more love than I even knew was possible. It's ironic that it took the near blindness that chemo caused to allow me to see this vision, to look at life more clearly than I ever had before.

At the time, I had no idea why I would be watching myself from behind walking up a ramp. At the time, I did not have much of an idea about anything. However, I do know I did hear a whisper that day as I walked up the ramp that I was going to beat cancer, and that happened before I was shown the vision. That is how I know it was of God. I know I was in the mirror, looking out at myself, seeing myself as God sees me. Knowing God's pure love of me allowed me to love myself as I had never before.

People always told her how strong she was, physically and mentally. She knew she had great strength. She felt invincible a lot. She wasn't sure where that strength came from but presumed her brain or stature were the likely reason for it. She was always grateful for it though and tried to teach it to others. The real hero of her story was finally found when there was little brain left and no brawn, just a scared woman in a broken body fighting for her next step and her life. It was then the Truth was revealed to her about where her real strength came from. Strength, the likes of which she had never had to call upon before, was only found through the grace of God's love. She was too sick to realize what was propelling her forward when it was all but impossible to move. Our patient God knew this and would wait for her to find this Truth in time. She now knows it was only the love of God that gave her the ability to push one leg in front of the other. It was His love that held her up when her body could not… His love that made her think she could when she couldn't think at all. He loves her, His child, and will do anything for her. He gave her life and gave her the strength and time to save her life.

Every time I now pause when seeing, hearing, thinking, or experiencing something, I know I am recognizing a message from God. I know that momentary stop in the flow of my day is to let me bookmark the image, words, or feelings so when they again come forward I will recognize that the lesson is ready to be revealed.

This next paragraph is what I was thinking as I was walking up the ramp, on my way to my chemo treatment, prior to the first time I had the vision of watching myself.

I was thinking about a fighter that I had seen on television when I was in high school. Our paths crossed as I was turning the channels looking for something to watch. I only stopped to watch his boxing match, which was nearing the end, because I was so taken aback by how bloody and severely beaten he was. I couldn't believe that, with all his wounds from the fight, he would continue to get up, over and over, and take another punch from his opponent. At that time, I couldn't comprehend why that fighter did that to himself. Why didn't he just lie down and concede the fight? Now, remembering this scene from over thirty years ago, I thought I knew what that man knew. I thought I had figured out that a true fighter gets up even when others' spirits would have been broken—rising, even when he knows that getting up again means another blow is coming. As I was walking, heading toward my next punch from chemo, against all odds of even standing, I thought I finally understood why a real fighter could never lay himself down for comfort or even out of necessity. After that, I heard the whisper that I would beat cancer. I did not know where it came from and was only able to hold on to the words long enough to get to my next gate.

Even though I never saw the fighter striking back at his opponent and I only saw him continuing to get up and stand before the next blow from his adversary hit him, I believed my thoughts were about fighting cancer. What I was actually seeing was the strength that the fighter received from God allowing him to not only rise, but stand from his Truth.

I now know from my Truth that sometimes the most honest part of the fight is when you can no longer compete with your human strength but stay in the ring anyway. When there is nothing left of everything that you thought you needed in order to win. When winning *Here* has been lost and you still find a way to again stand inside the ring from *Over There.* Maybe the constriction of the ropes allows you to find the courage to hold on by letting go, and to rise from your Truth. Maybe that's when you understand that God is your real strength, providing not just the will, but also the means to get up over and over. Maybe that's why some get up and others don't. Some call upon God, and others forget His name. Maybe that's why everyone roots for the underdog. They cheer for him because they know that if he can find strength greater than his human capacity—God—at that moment, even what looks like a loss is really the greatest victory. And sometimes when the odds are beat and the impossible is achieved, letting the *less than* become more than enough to win, everyone applauds and rejoices. Not because of the score but from the unspoken knowing of everyone watching the fight: that God was there and He was the reason for the victory.

There is not enough love in this human world to love you out of your mind's thinking that you are unlovable. God's infinite love for you will overwhelm your mind's unlovingness. Once you feel God's love, it knocks down the human barrier your mind has cemented between you and love. You can then begin to accept love from anyone or anywhere, and fill your heart with the fullness of life's gifts.

When your heart is hurt by your mind repeatedly throughout your life, a chasm is formed from the wounds created by your mind's false beliefs about you. This chasm sits between your heart and God. When you do not heal these cuts, no matter how small, they keep burrowing into your heart further and deeper. After a while, too many little hurts grow too big. You could have a thousand small gashes or one big one, but either way you have moved away from God. The only way to heal your injuries is from love. Too often, people who have been hurt too much, even if it's from their own mind, don't know how to let in healing love. That is why their wounds are unable to heal. When your heart is broken, it can lose its ability to accept love, as your broken heart feels unworthy. And even at precious times when your heart is able to let love in, you may not have the ability to find that love within it again.

One of the thoughts I had in one of my *How did I get cancer* moments was that in the preceding year, before I got sick, my youngest son was no longer cuddling with me all the time like when he was younger. Both of my boys were more independent now and running around with their friends. I was happy that they were self-confident enough to do so. However, I also remember at the same time that my heart really missed that physical connection and continuous flow of abundant love they gave me. It was like an intravenous drug pumped directly into my heart that sometimes I felt a little addicted to. I wondered if maybe that love was keeping my broken heart on life support and now that its flow had decreased with my kids getting older, I allowed my hurt to become too big.

The other side of that thought was knowing that I still had somehow been able to find enough of that love to hold on to when I had been on the ropes during chemo. The love of my boys would well up in me and grow every time things got worse. All the past love I had in my heart is what kept me alive during the worst crises of my cancer treatment. I knew their love for me and my love for them was what gave me the strength to live. What I did not know at that time was that all of the love that my kids had given me over the years, and all of the love that I had given to them had remained in my heart. I just didn't know how to access it and I kept thinking it was gone as soon as the moment was over. When I was too sick for my *less than* mind to keep me from God, I could access this love from my Truth when I needed it the most in order to live. After I got through the storm, I would have no idea how it happened and could no longer find it because I again let my mind take control. Once I learned how to hold on to God, I could heal my heart and feel that love every day through my Truth.

You must now face toward the light to feel as much warmth from love as you can.

Cancer treatment is extra hard on someone whose cancer is caused by their broken heart. Cancer isolates you, further removing you from the love you so desperately need. The after effects of chemo, surgery, and radiation seal off your body from physical contact in a thousand different ways and stop the flow of the critical love that you need. In addition to your time away from your family for treatment, your body is in so much pain that you have to pull yourself back from physical human contact that you previously took for granted. Your body is on such high alert that every touch or sensation can send shooting sparks of pain through you. I was in so much discomfort that I could not bear to even have my clothes touching me. This meant my husband had to sleep on the couch since even the slightest movement of our mattress bothered me. It also meant that I could no longer let my kids on my bed in the morning to snuggle as we used to do every day before cancer. Just hugging my kids as I always loved to do was now only done in the moments where they really needed it and I could endure the pain it caused. I had to find new ways to get the love I needed to heal my heart.

Once I started feeling God's love for me and later feeling that kind of love for myself, I was able to fully accept love from people other than my husband and children. I was able, for the first time, to fill in my hearts wounds left by cancer as well as the holes that had been open long before that.

My sister Linda called me as soon as Mom told her I had breast cancer. Her deep compassion and concern for me and her openness to share with me how she overcame her own health issues years earlier, deeply touched me. When she called and told me that she had a business trip to Chicago and wanted to spend an extra day there to be with me during my second chemo, I couldn't believe it. She was going out of her way for me. I never asked or expected anyone, even my sister, to use their valuable time for me without my having earned it or intending to pay them back. It meant so much that she wanted to do that for me. That I was important enough to her that she would take time from her busy life just for me. She did it a second time too for another one of my chemos. She came to be with me, and that meant the world to me—someone who wouldn't even take her own time for herself.

My neighbor Jo from across the street gave me the steady love I so desperately needed as I was surrounded by chaos. She would pop over and check on me, and when she noticed I was gone for a few days she would bring over home-cooked food for my family. Jo served as my ambassador to cancer survival, sharing with me her story of breast cancer from over a decade earlier. She candidly and calmly spoke of her experiences so that I could know that, although difficult, there was an ending to the ordeal and a long future life was possible. Her love and quiet calmness and composure through her cancer was a beautiful example of how to find mine.

Other people, like my son's friend's mom, Amy, whom I had only known from dropping off and picking up my son at play dates and activities, showed up too. This caring woman would write long handwritten notes in cards for me, encouraging me to stay strong, telling me that I would make it through and that she was there to help. I was so overwhelmed that she even took the time to go out and buy me a card and drop it off at my house, let alone write these beautiful notes of reassurance. Her cards were always impeccably timed too; just when I needed a little extra love or reassurance, they would show up. Sometimes when they did and I was too sick to open them for a few days; I would just stare at them, knowing that she cared about me.

I also had many people's love brought to me through prayer circles. This was the first time I began to understand the amazing providence of people brought together by their love of God to access the power of God through prayer. I couldn't believe it as I watched people constantly doing things for me that I had never thought to do for myself. They did it because they knew everyone is worthy of God's love and knew they could bring me God's love and healing through prayer.

One day I ventured outside of my house after a couple of days of, oddly, feeling a bit better. My next-door neighbor Pebble saw me and came over to see how I was doing. While we were talking about how I was feeling, she told me that she had her prayer group praying for me that week. I didn't even know she was religious, let alone in a prayer group. This was the third time that someone had told me that they had put me in their prayer group—and, prior to my knowing it was happening, I had noticed a slight improvement in my state. I know that with illness there are ebbs and flows to the days; some days you feel better and some days you don't. But I somehow knew that day, the third time it happened as a coincidence, that it was the prayers that made the difference. Because I now knew there were no such things as coincidences; only divine order. I was blessed to have people who knew God in a way that I, as yet, did not, praying for me.

I was supported and prayed for by too many family and friends to list. My cousin, Amy, even ran a race for breast cancer in my honor. I was offered love by all of these people, and for the first time, I fully accepted it, knowing I was worthy of it. Because I was now standing with God and not in my *less than* mind, I was able to receive their love as it was given freely and purely, knowing nothing was expected in return. It was by watching people whom I loved love me, and people whom I didn't even know love me that I began to figure out that I was not *less than* and good enough to receive their love. It was this love, this abundance of pure love, that helped heal my broken heart and lift me out of the *less than* pit I had fallen into. These people were not only important in making the difference in my healing but for showing me the simple, beautiful power of love and prayer.

If you are not able to be around me in peace and love, then I can only know you from a distance. I now love myself too much to let someone else's pain and judgments drain my life force to serve their needs.

While I was opening up more to all the beautiful people bringing me love when I was sick, I also had to put space between me and people who were in wounding judgment of me and could hurt my heart. I didn't do it to be vindictive or point a finger, accusing them of harming me. I did it because I knew that, if I wanted to live, I could not take in anything other than love. I did it because negativity and judgments were even more painful now that I did not have the strength most days to lift my *more than* shield to protect myself. The only thing I could do was put a physical distance between their harmful energy and me. This meant that anyone who was not of pure love and acceptance of me was not allowed in our house. It was not forever. It was until I had my strength back and could either sort it out with them or part ways for good. I had to put an emergency moratorium into effect and keep out anyone from my life who brought with them anything other than love for me.

I am now much more sensitive to other people's negativity and judgments toward me, or anyone, or anything else. I do not like to be around it in any shape or form if I can help it. Many people I know who have had cancer feel as I do. I think that is for two reasons: One, although everyone can sense how negative energy hijacks their physical energy, that sense gets heightened when you are in survival mode and you intuitively know it is life-threatening to further drain your life force. And two, when you are sick and want to get better, you have no choice but to dump anything that is not positive, because it's just too heavy to carry in your heart. Once you release the weight of your own, as well as other people's false assessments and disapproval, you feel so much lighter and more alive. You then become much more aware of and sensitive to the burden and uncomfortable feeling that harmful judgment brings to your body.

Some of the seemingly benign moments, passing thoughts, and random experiences turned out to be much more than that. They were beautiful reminders of God.

"God writes the gospel not in the Bible alone, but also in the trees, and in the flowers and clouds and stars." Martin Luther

My husband and I had talked about buying a boat for years. However, we always decided to put it off until we were done remodeling, until we moved, until the kids got older, until we had enough money, until we had the time—but it was actually just until I got cancer. Yes, cancer is the reason we bought our pontoon. Right in the middle of being sick, during the last three months of my chemo, we bought a boat. When you are facing your mortality, you get around to the *untils* faster than planned. It turned out to be impeccable timing. I would get my weekly Taxol chemo on Thursdays, so I had until Sunday, thanks to the steroids, before I crashed and burned. Saturdays could go either way… and they did. Nevertheless, no matter what, we went out on the boat every Saturday. We went even if I was sick, because there was something about the time on the pontoon that made life easier for all of us. I would always feel better both physically and mentally on the boat. I think it was from the rocking motion of the boat as it rested on the water.

I always admired the ability of ships to float. Science was not my strong suit in school, but anytime I heard about the buoyancy of vessels, I admired its genius. Even in first grade, when I learned about Columbus, I thought it was amazing that ships could carry all those people and sail all the way from Spain to America. I was more impressed with the Nina, the Pinta, and the Santa Maria than with Columbus. The ability to remain afloat and always seek balance, which is what boats and ships do, is a beautiful and majestic thing to me. If the waves are high, boats seemed to instinctively know just how swiftly to rock, seeking their balance. If the water is calm, they only move just enough to maintain their equilibrium.

Sitting or lying on the pontoon helped remind not just my mind but also my body of the pureness of buoyancy, and the sacredness of balancing a man-made object in the water of life. It seemed that as soon as we pushed off from the dock, away from the land, my entire family found their balance and was able to take a deep breath and relax. Everything that was happening was left on shore, and we floated with ease and peace for the next three or four hours. Every night when we came back home, I could still feel the relaxing motion of the boat rocking inside of my body, providing balance and a calming peace to my body, even as the chemo was ravaging it. I love our pontoon and what it gave to me. It was worth every penny we still owe on it, and more.

I believe in angels and I know they walk amongst us. They become visible when you are with God. That is when you can see through their cloak and are aware of their light.

The fifth round of the A/C Red Devil shrank my tumor again. The orange-sized tissue attempting to encapsulate my tumor disappeared, and the size of my tumor felt substantially smaller too. I did not opt for the sixth round of A/C, as the *more-chemo* doctor suggested, deciding instead that the A/C did its magic and that my heart probably had had enough of the Red Devil. I then went on to complete six of my twelve weekly installments of Taxol chemo—and, surprise, surprise, I felt the tumor beginning to grow again. I went back to Chicago and told them I thought it was time to stop the Taxol and do surgery, as I felt it sprouting again. The physician's assistant said she thought it felt bigger too, and the doctor agreed to order a mammogram to see if it was indeed expanding. The test showed that the tumor had shrunk about thirty percent from the size it was when it was encapsulated within the orange-sized uprising in my breast.

I knew that this shrinkage happened within two weeks of the fifth A/C treatment, before I started the Taxol. At that time, I had requested a test so we would know how much the tumor had decreased before I started the unknown Taxol, so that if it wasn't working I could know and would stop taking it. My cancer sheep request was denied. Now, when I was six weeks into the Taxol, the test they ran of course showed the tumor was reduced in size. I explained twenty-five ways to Sunday to the physician's assistant, who then kept relaying my pleas to the doctor: that, yes, it was smaller than before the orange, but it was the A/C that had reduced it, not the Taxol. Now it was growing again since the Taxol was not working. Still, the doctor refused to believe me and would not budge on her decision that it was the Taxol, not the A/C, that had shrunk the tumor.

So I did it again; I kept doing the chemo because no one would listen to someone whom they believed knew less about her body than they did. I now know I never stood a chance against that doctor in Chicago, even at the beginning, because I was in fear and she was on her home court. I didn't understand how to play the game of cancer, and the chemo quickly took away my mental and physical ability to win any contest against her. It is hard enough to cure cancer, but to have the person leading the charge not listening to you stacks the odds against you even higher. I am no longer mad at her, but still disappointed that when I most needed someone to protect me, she choose to fight me. I was vulnerable and needed someone to listen to what I knew about my body, not to stand on her medical degree and dismiss me. At one of my appointments, when I was one of the last patients being seen for the day, I watched everyone in the doctor's office getting ready to leave. This is when I realized that everyone who works in the doctor's office or hospital gets to go home every night and step away from cancer. We, the patients, did not. We went home with our cancer and what was—or was not—given to us to help. My hope is that more doctors become open to understanding that they do not know everything and everyone like a textbook. Cancer is one of the most confounding diseases to medicine. If you press most doctors, you will quickly get to the speech that "no one really knows how to cure cancer." That's why it is so necessary that doctors be open to hearing what those who have it are telling them… that is where they may find an opening and the miracle to cure it.

I reluctantly did three more weeks of Taxol. When I went in for my tenth round of Taxol in Fargo, I could barely walk. Even the steroids that day could not make me believe I had any energy. I now know that the false energy of the steroids is what convinced me that I was strong enough to keep doing chemo. I also could not focus my eyes, as the Taxol had affected my optical nerves. As I sat in the chair getting ready to have them poke my port, hoping they could draw blood so they could then inject me with more chemo, I started crying. I was by then used to crying a lot, but this time I just could not stop. I knew I could not let one more drop of that poison enter my body. I became inconsolable, causing the nurse to almost cry with me. She told me that she could not administer the chemo to me if I was this upset and that unsure about getting it.

The one thing that I quickly came to realize during my cancer treatment was that the nurses in my story were really angels—every single one of them, without exception. I believe people who choose to be nurses are angels here on earth. They are the real heroes of our world, and until you are sick, you cannot comprehend their grace. I never had a nurse—and I had many of them—who wasn't caring. The nurses during my MRSA diarrhea, who, every time I apologized, told me they didn't care how many times they had to change my dirty sheets; or the nurse who fought everyone to get me better anti-nausea meds before she gave me antibiotics so I wouldn't throw up; or this nurse who held my hand and cared more about me than the chemo. That nurse found a way to have a doctor sign off on a $300 sonogram to see if the tumor had shrunk in the last three weeks since my last test in Chicago. It had not. Again I knew what I knew, and so did that nurse. I went home that day knowing that I would never do chemo again—saving Blue Cross and Blue Shields thousands on the unused chemo and finally saving me from that doctor in Chicago who refused to listen to me.

It is one thing to feel afraid as you watch yourself in a nightmare when you are asleep. It is even scarier to watch yourself in real life as you are living in your nightmare.

You are required to wait three weeks after you stop chemo before you can have surgery. Due to the surgeons' schedule, I was going to have to wait almost four. Although the tumor was growing back, I was still grateful for the delay. Though I had stopped chemo, I still felt like I was on it. I was even more tired now since I was not taking the steroids to have me believe differently. Those last three weeks of chemo had taken such a toll on the nerves in my feet and eyes as well as my energy that I did not think my body was coming back this time. When I had first started chemo, it took a week to recover; now it was almost four, and I was not sure I would ever regain my strength. I didn't know if my eyesight would return or if I would ever again be able to do more than shuffle my feet to get places. I sat there knowing how physically weak I was, understanding the risk of keeping the growing tumor in me every day. I was facing a six-hour surgery and not sure if I would wake up from it. This is the meaning of "a rock and a hard place."

I wanted to make a video for my sons in case I didn't make it through my surgery. Remembering their lonely faces that day when I was in the hospital with MRSA, I did not want to leave them without something to hold on to. Having to read my kids a letter that they would read after my death was probably one of the worst parts of my whole nightmare. I read the letter in front of our video camera that sat precariously on an unstable camera stand I had found at a garage sale. My husband and I tried many takes until I was able to just cry a little, not the entire way through. I ended up looking and sounding like the broken woman I was, trying to beg her sons for forgiveness for leaving them.

As I sat there, incapable of delivering what were potentially my last words to my sons, I remembered how many times Dan had told me how much he loved listening to me on my work conference calls. Hearing my words and how knowledgeable I was. Feeling the energy my voice contained as I came up with solutions and designs for my customers. Listening to the solidness and sureness of my proposals. Seeing my smile and how I was genuine and could make people laugh. I now spoke, not knowing about anything, especially tomorrow. I was out of ideas, hunched over and crying, not having heard my *confidence* in months. All that remained was my shame as I clumsily mouthed my words through overwhelming desperation and discomfort, unable to even assure my sons that it would be all right if I weren't there anymore. My speech was delivered from the depths and darkness of my *less than* chasm. I knew that if they watched that video after I died they would watch knowing that the woman speaking those words was not their mother. They would know that I had been long gone before that woman even finished her first sentence. I still have the video but have not watched it since the day I made it. I don't think I will ever watch it again, because that sad, broken, *less than* woman no longer needs to speak for me.

Thunks in the night were no longer as terrifying or as uncommon to me as they used to be.

Two days before I was scheduled to leave for my lumpectomy, in the middle of the night, the screws fell out of my bedroom closet system of shelves and rods that held my clothes. We had lived in our house for a little over two years at that point, and those same clothes had sat on the shelves and hung on the rods from the first day. I had not touched any of the clothes in that closet since I had been sick since most of them were for work and dressing up. When I heard the noise, it woke me up, but I was so tired I just rolled over and fell back asleep. The next morning I didn't even bother to worry about what the noise could have been. However, the next day before I was to leave for my surgery and went to pack, I opened up the closet door to get my suitcase and I saw all of my clothes lying on the floor. I thought I now understood what all the noise was about.

At first I didn't want to deal with the mess since I was tired and had to fly to Chicago the next day. My first thought was to just leave it all there until I got back from my surgery. Then an overwhelming desire came upon me to throw everything out. I wanted all those clothes gone. I felt like I could no longer wear those clothes. I also could not, for some reason, leave them lying there until I got back. I then considered having my husband clean them up for me while I was gone. However, my resistance to that idea was overpowering, feeling that I needed to go through every piece myself and get rid of everything today! So I filled up six big, black garbage bags with my best clothes that I had accumulated over the last twenty years. My current work clothes, dress-up clothes, my fat clothes, my skinny clothes, my clothes that I kept for nostalgia and never intended to wear again, along with the clothes I bought but never found an occasion to wear. *All* of them. They needed to go, and they did. It took all day and a couple of naps in between, but I could not leave them lying there until I got back. I had no idea why the day before I went to have a lumpectomy I decided to throw out the last twenty years of what provided cover for my life. I also had no idea that in a couple of days I was also going to throw out my breasts too.

Letting go of things that you never intended to let go of is easier than you know in the moment, and harder to grasp later on. Nevertheless, either way, it has been done and should never be regretted, because the opened space can be refilled with love.

My mom joined me in Chicago for my lumpectomy surgery. I had researched all my choices and options and knew that triple-negative is no more likely to return in the breast if you have a lumpectomy than a mastectomy, making a lumpectomy a sufficient choice. Since day one, I never considered having a mastectomy. However, something happened as I was going through all the pre-op tests and evaluations. I don't know why, but I suddenly decided that I wanted a mastectomy. *Wait… what… WHAT? We're not cutting off our breasts. The left one is fine. Is It? How do you know? How do you know it is not in other places in the right one too?*

I did this desperate, barbaric act to myself because I knew at that point that the chemo had been a miserable failure. It was a crushing lose that topped all my past defeats in life combined. Chemo just did not perform as advertised. My odds of living life going forward were far less than a coin toss, so I chose to do something to myself more brutal than injecting poison. I cut off my breasts. I did not do it bravely; I did it out of the fear of knowing the chemo did not work—

the panic of knowing that medicine had nothing left in its bag of tricks for me. Maybe I wanted to wipe the slate clean so I could start again. Maybe I simply made the choice that nothing fit anymore, including my breasts.

I was told that, along with the mastectomy, they were going to remove ten to twelve lymph nodes since I had at least one affected node. It turned out they removed seventeen. It always seemed that the plans made before treatment inevitably ended up taking more from me than promised. So there I was with four drainage tubes sticking out of my sides and unable to lift my now numb right arm, looking like a twelve-year-old boy.

God showed me that lambs of God do not need to flinch when sheep speak.

Everyone told me to tell my children I had cancer. I did not feel like putting a name on what was happening to me *and* them. It was clear to them I was ill. When I told them I was sick, my son Sam actually asked if I had cancer. He quickly followed that question up by telling me he knew a kid whose grandpa had cancer and died. This confirmed my decision to not say the word. I knew that I could not have any type of conversation telling them to not worry about me having cancer. I couldn't say, "I'm going to live even though someone's grandpa died," because I did not know that to be true. I would not take the chance of having my kids catch me in the biggest lie of my life.

People were very persistent in telling me that I was wrong not to tell my sons I had cancer. I was told that children are resilient and given books about how to tell them mommy has cancer. I read them cover to cover searching for a reason why I should, but never found one. I finally just started telling people that I would not tell my boys that I had cancer any more than I would tell them Santa Claus was not real. I was not going to break my children's hearts with the most terrifying word in the world: *cancer*—unless I knew for sure that death was inevitable or living was for sure. I was going to allow my sons to have as much happiness as long as they could without imposing the name of my pain in their lives. Even if it were one more day without having to know that word, it would be one more day they could live without the burden of the word *cancer.* Knowing that I was now defined by that word, I was not going to let them anywhere near it if possible. Being a bad mom in the eyes of the world because I would not give my kids the unreturnable gift of the word *cancer* was one more thing I put in the *less than* chasm with me to drag along through my nightmare.

Shortly after I stopped chemo, I again flew to Chicago. Now, as I entered the limo and again became a rock star, I removed my baseball cap and fake hair halo piece. There is no denying your cancer when you have rock star status. I always flew in late for my appointments, and when I arrived at the hotel, I would be exhausted. On this night, as I was carrying my bag into the hotel to check in, I somehow dropped my baseball cap and hair in the lobby.

The next morning, when I got up, I could not find them and was running late, so I went to the hospital without cover, owning my rock star status. I was no longer completely bald, but my hair was thin and short, like a kid's crew cut at the beginning of summer. I would not walk around at home like that, but there it was not uncommon to see a sheared sheep.

After returning from my appointments that night, I asked the hotel front desk if they had found my head gear, and they had. I surprised myself when I was getting ready to go home the next day; I decided not to wear them. Truthfully, my hair was still too short to pass as a person who did not have cancer. I was slightly uncomfortable about the state of my head, but for the first time I just did not want to wear the hair and hat that day, so I decided to wear a bit of make-up to compensate for my hair shortfall. As I walked through the airport and people looked oddly at me, I just kept saying to myself that they just didn't understand how hip and cosmopolitan I am to wear my hair so short.

When I took my seat on the airplane, a young man in his late twenties sat down next to me and smiled as we exchanged hellos. I do not know why, but I asked him, "Do you like my haircut?" He politely said, "Yes," then followed up, telling me that it was a little short for his taste but kindly said it looked good on me. For some reason at that point, I stopped being hip and cosmopolitan and got brave, telling him it was growing back from chemo. I *never* talked to people on planes about my cancer, fearing that after people knew my secret they would become uncomfortable around me, or tell me they knew someone who died from it, or, worse yet, pity me. I had seen one too many "oh, that poor woman" gazes for a lifetime.

Nevertheless, today I told this young man I had cancer—the last person I would have expected to want me to share that piece of information. But as it turned out he was the exact right person to tell my secret. He immediately told me his mom had breast cancer when he was ten. I shared with him that one of my sons was ten when I got sick. He continued to talk more about the time when his mom had cancer. He said that before his mother got sick, his family was really close and did everything together. However, when she went to the hospital for treatment, they would not tell him why she had to go there. He said that at the time he was mad and hurt because his parents had never kept secrets from him before, and he felt left out. *Ahhh.* I thought he was going to tell me something I didn't want to hear. Another something I got all wrong. I had not yet told him that I also was keeping this same secret from my sons. I decided that, before telling him this, I wanted to hear from him whether being mad at your parents for not telling you about your mom's cancer and feeling left out was worse than knowing your mom had cancer. I asked him, "Now that you're twenty-seven, do you think that they did the right thing by not telling you?"

It was as if I was sitting next to my grown son in seventeen years' time and asking if I made the right choice. I had no idea what his response would be. The foreboding, "Dant-dant-da!" moment became anticlimactic when he said that he now understood why they made the decision to not tell him. I needed more and asked him, "Even though you now understand why they didn't tell you, do you think it would have been better if they had told you the truth?" In a second more breathtaking and not at all foreboding, "Dant-dant-da!" moment he went on to say that if he could go back and tell them what to do, he would have told them to not tell him about her cancer. He said he was now glad that he did not know what was wrong with his mom. Knowing it was cancer would have been too scary and worse than being mad and feeling left out. What are the odds of having that conversation with a now grown man who, as a ten-year-old boy, had a mother with breast cancer who did not tell him? Just as I was not telling my ten- and seven-year-olds. And what's more, he thought that his parents did the right thing. That is not random. That is God putting people in your life, offering you what you need to hear. I now know why I didn't want to wear my hat and hair that day. After I got off the plane, I did not go hat- and hair-free again for another two months.

Now, as the physical pain was receding the tide came in, allowing the waves of mental pain further onto the shore.

"Forgive, sounds good. Forget, I'm not sure I could. They say time heals everything. But I'm still waiting. I'm through with doubt. There's nothing left for me to figure out. I've paid a price, and I'll keep paying. I'm not ready to make nice. I'm not ready to back down. I'm still mad as hell, and I don't have time to go round and round and round. It's too late to make it right. I probably wouldn't if I could. Cause I'm mad as hell. Can't bring myself to do what it is you think I should. I know you said can't you just get over it? It turned my whole world around and I kinda like it. I made my bed, and I sleep like a baby. With no regrets." Not Ready to Make Nice -Dixie Chicks

Four weeks after surgery, I was scheduled to begin radiation. I was going to do it at the happiest place on earth, but the magic show was much less intoxicating in Chicago now. Instead, I chose to drive the 180 miles round trip to Fargo every day Monday through Friday for radiation.

My radiation treatments started just before Thanksgiving, right in the midst of the North Dakota winter. At times the weather and road conditions were so bad I had to stay in a hotel in Fargo because driving was impossible. Most days, though, I drove back and forth in the subzero temperatures, blowing snow, and icy roads. I thought it would be too pathetically ironic at that point, after everything I had gone through, to end up dying in a traffic accident. So I felt reasonably safe driving in semi-blizzard conditions.

Driving in that weather was like my deepest days of chemo. I watched the snow whipping around in the North Dakota wind and blowing across the road, taunting my car, many times blinding me to what was right in front of me on the other side of the windshield. It was during this time, when my focus was on the narrow amount of visible inches in front of me, that I would process the memories of the previous nine months. I learned how to stop holding my breath and to breathe through them, just as I was breathing through the snowstorm. I would concentrate on staying on the road and just rhythmically inhaling the storm and exhaling the pain.

On the days when the weather took a break, I would change my tactics to release my grief. I would sing the Dixie Chicks song, "I'm Not Ready to Make Nice" over and over, always at the top of my lungs, many times screaming more than singing, sometimes crying. I had to get it all out, every bit of the pain. There were many, many miles between Fargo and Jamestown. I used every one of them to drive out and let go of my pain.

I did not think radiation was really going to help my cause. After knowing that chemo hadn't worked on my tumor, let alone my body, which was much more important to cleanse, I wasn't sure what the point was of radiating my now nonexistent breast. I still decided to go forward with the remainder of the poison-cut-and-burn trifecta, thinking that if cancer came back I would at least be able to tell my kids I did everything possible to prevent it. I also knew it wouldn't cause as much damage to my body as the chemo. I thought, *What the heck. Let's finish strong.* However, shortly after I started, I felt like I didn't want to keep doing it. I didn't know why I but could not bring myself to stop. I just kept going. I just would not pull the plug on it. My friend Sandi told me to pray to God about whether I should stop. I did, but I never heard anything back so I compromised with myself and decided that I was just going to do it until I completed thirty—not thirty-five treatments.

In six weeks I completed twenty-six treatments and had every intention of getting all thirty done. It was a week before Christmas, and I woke up on Sunday morning thinking I had had a really strange dream. I had heard a woman telling me, "It's over. You're okay now." I was half asleep and yet somehow half awake. I was having a conversation with the female voice, telling her that I could not believe what she was saying. I went on to tell her that I could not trust my intuition or whoever she was because of my words that were so wrong about cancer that day in the doctor's office, the day when the nurse was scheduling me for a mammogram. I told her that I was sorry and that, even though I would like to believe her, I could not. My intuition had lied to me before, and I could not trust it. Then I heard her kind voice through her eternal patience, speaking to my endless doubts. She simply said, "You were not wrong in what you thought or what you said to that nurse. Cancer will not take you out. You never said you wouldn't get cancer; you only said that it would not take you out. I'm here to tell you that you were right. You can trust yourself and what you know to be true. You can believe the words that often fall from your mouth before you can catch them to hide their Truth. These words come from a voice that knows you from beyond this world." By now I was wide awake as her words trailed off.

Wait... what... WHAT? I was in shock. I had just spent the last ten months thinking my intuition was dead wrong and that I could no longer trust it. The gestation cycle was complete and I was now reborn, awakened from my heroic-coma dream-turned-nightmare. Now understanding what I had forgotten, not just about God, but His voice. Realizing I had known everything I needed to know in order to heal all along, but couldn't escape my mind to hold on and remember how. I now remembered who I was and where God was.

At that point, I still had a deep fog of chemo brain and could not understand a simple knock-knock joke. I certainly did not have the capacity to come up with what the kind and patient voice had just told me about my words not lying. How she clarified my words and came up with an explanation of what my words meant was miraculous. I had spent ten months lamenting over those words, and that voice had explained their Truth—cancer was not going to take me out, which my human mind was incapable of understanding.

Whenever I experience God, I always feel the most amazing and endless patience; unlimited tranquility that contains only love. When the female voice talked with me in my dream, I knew it was not from my mind because of her comforting patience with me; calmness I did not know then how to have with myself.

I did not go back to radiation the week before Christmas, because of what the voice told me. The following Monday, after the radiation department had left several messages, I called them and told them I would not be coming back. They asked if I would come in and discuss my decision with the doctor. Knowing that the radiologist had treated me well, I decided it was the right thing to do. My radiologist was one of the best doctors I encountered during my treatments. In our first meeting, he shared that he had read my entire cancer history and acknowledged that I had been through a lot. He was both knowledgeable and professional. He answered all of my questions and was forthright with any information he shared with me. He, however, had something that had been missing from my other encounters with the cancer gods. He had an open heart. I was treated as an individual, not a cancer sheep; like an equal, not a *less than.* I did not feel like a badge with a name and the letter (P) for patient notated beside it, but a friend or a sister for whom he wanted to do his best.

Even knowing this, I still was not sure what I was going to tell him since I did not want him to judge me or God. After sitting down and again feeling that he respected me enough to listen and would be open to what he heard, I told him what I was told by the female voice of God. In the big "*Dant-dant-da!*" moment, I held my breath, unsure of what was going to come back at me. After experiencing much more disrespect from doctors for much less provocative statements than this, he told me that he would never judge what happens between someone and God. It wasn't lip service; he meant it and was kind and reverent to God when he said it. I am not sure if he believed what I said actually happened or if he thought I was some mentally exhausted woman who had had enough of the cancer parade. But it didn't matter either way because he honored what I said. He did not dismiss it out of hand as had been done so many times to me before. He told me he would respect my decision and reviewed my options: quitting altogether, doing four more to complete what I had initially planned, or doing four more and then a week of booster radiation.

I decided to do the remaining four dosages, which was my original plan. He told me that in the future, when I looked back, I would be glad that I did them. I somehow believed his statement, but I knew it was not for the same reasons he did. At first I thought it would give me four more days to drive out the memories of the past ten months. I was now singing the Dixie Chicks song, "I Believe in Love." Even though I did cherish my time driving, and it was part of the reason I chose to do four more treatments, I later figured out it was not the true reason.

"... Silence stared me in the face. And I finally heard its voice. It seemed to softly say that in love you have choice. Today I got the answer. And there's a world of truth behind it. Love is out there waiting somewhere. You just have to go and find it. I believe in love, I believe in love. A love that's real, love that's strong. Love that lives on and on. Yes I believe in love. Yes I believe in love." I Believe In Love -Dixie Chicks.

I wasn't sure how I was going to feel doing four more treatments. I didn't know if I was going to feel like I was betraying the voice of God or if I would be thinking, *Phew, I'm glad I did this because it will make me feel more protected and keep me from fearing the future.* When I was again lying under the machine for my treatment, I found my answer. My Truth allowed me to know that radiation did not make one bit of difference because I was healed. Lying there during my last four treatments allowed me to experience and understand the steadfast knowing of my Truth. During each of those five-minute radiation zaps, I lay within my Truth, knowing I was healed.

I know now why it's okay to not know the reason you sometimes do things. When you are compelled to do something, even when you think you don't want to yet you have peace while doing it, you are honoring your Truth. Just because I did not need to do the radiation because my cancer was healed did not mean it wasn't necessary to do the radiation for other healing reasons. This was the first time since I had been sick that I received treatment without fear. I began to realize that something else was happening to me alongside the outward act of getting radiation that was healing me. Maybe the whole time, all the chemo, surgery, and radiation was the mirage of a cure, that allowed me to go to places inside of me where the real healing needed to take place.

Maybe in a roundabout way, the chemo, surgery, and radiation did heal me. Maybe it wasn't the actual trifecta but the terrible side effects of chemo, the letting go from the surgery, and the long drives to radiation along with all the people and circumstances I met through my cancer journey that made the magic happen. After all, my Truth was that I needed to heal my heart by healing my mind, and all my other healing would flow from that. Maybe what happened to me was not at all what it seemed.

Maybe I didn't know what I didn't know, and what I went through happened exactly the way it should so that I would find a way to the other side of my heart, to find God and heal my cancer. Learning how to find peace and experiencing a love greater than I had ever known only happened after poisoning, cutting, and burning false parts of my mind that hid the most important part of me: God. Unknown to me, God was surging through my heart beneath my breast along with the chemo, and radiation. Maybe it took the chemicals in the chemo and rays in the radiation to light up God in order for me to see Him. Therefore, I needed those last four radiations—but not for the reasons one would think. Those last four radiation treatments taught me that it was the needle of man's medicine that was able to show me the hand of God. So all that I went through was exactly as it needed to be. The peace of knowing that was worth a few tanks of gas.

That's who Sandi is. Someone who showed me that you should not be afraid to announce any of your Truths to anyone. Sandi knows Truth is worthy of a voice. The voice of Truth can carry messages out to those who need to hear them most. The most important Truth she ever shared with me was that we no longer had cancer. She was residing in her Truth and showed me how to stand in mine. I love you, Sandi, my sister.

God gave me Sandi. I met her a couple of months into my treatments. I was once again sitting in the atrium of the hospital in Chicago. It was never lost on me that the most healing things that happened to me in that place happened in the atrium, not in the medical treatment rooms. Maybe that was where the true magic show was going on, because I sure found God there a lot.

I was in an "I'm not talking to anyone" mood and sitting back in my green reclining chair, resting and waiting for the shuttle to take me back to my hotel when I noticed a woman standing near me with a beautiful, shimmering, red-and-black scarf on her head. I noted that she had on dark lipstick and bold eye makeup, and I thought, *Good for her.* I didn't have the right attitude to put extra effort into myself like that. She saw me looking at her. Since she was standing close enough to me, I broke my rule of silence and told her I liked her scarf. She then opened up and began talking to me. You could see her light brightly shining within her. Yes, she too had breast cancer.

Looks were not deceiving. It turned out that Sandi was the most put-together person with cancer that I have ever met. She knew her healing was preordained and she just needed to walk through her treatment. She owned her *recovery*, not the cancer. Sandi did not focus on her tough medical breaks; she only gave conversation space to what she was going to do next. We became instant friends and happened to be staying at the same hotel. After riding the shuttle to our hotel, we sat in the lobby and talked and talked. We then went out nearby the hotel and walked around a quaint antique shop and got something to eat. Later we talked into the night in her hotel room, as if we had been friends for years. I felt like I was back in college hanging out in my friend's dorm room. I met my new BFF, breast friend forever, on a day I didn't plan to talk to anyone.

Sandi was about two months ahead of me in her treatments. She not only helped me understand what was next on my cancer to-do list, but also was someone who knew exactly what I was going through. I could share things with her that other people just could not stomach about cancer, like what it does to your body and mind. She brought me such comfort and immediately invited me into her big world. I told her about my heart guard, and she told me that she too had to protect her heart now more than ever. When I shared my disappointments with myself, she shared hers with me. She then told me to let it go; we were just doing the best we could. We only needed to be grateful that we knew better now.

She knew about everything I was just beginning to wonder about. She would explain all about organics, supplements, and life. Most importantly, she began teaching me more about God. I had never read the Bible, but she knew it chapter and verse. She stood proud and firm in her relationship with God, and she shared her beliefs with me, freely speaking, without hesitation, of God's greatness and His love. She was the human hand of God I could hold as I was walking through cancer. We walked side by side with each other and God for our ups, downs, setbacks, and triumphs. From that point forward, we would always try to book our appointments so that we would be at the hospital at the same time. At our last cancer rendezvous, Sandi announced my freedom from cancer. She repeated the words out loud that I had heard only a few short weeks earlier from the voice in my dream.

It was the beginning of January and we had both completed our chemo and our mastectomies. She was at the hospital to continue her reconstructive surgery, and I was there for my end-of-treatment checkup. Sandi and I were sitting next to each other on the shuttle, going back to the hotel after dinner at the hospital and talking with other cancer travelers. After someone had finished sharing their cancer story with us, the inevitable next question came. "What cancer do you two have?" Sandi replied, without missing a beat, "Oh, we don't have cancer anymore!" I almost fell out of my seat. I had told others about what the voice had said in my dream; I had even had that same conversation with myself during my last four radiations—but I had never said those words out loud as my Truth. Somehow, hearing

Sandi's announcement to everyone on the shuttle about our cancer status, through her unfaltering voice, made my words real. And that was that… we were out of the cancer club. Sandi turned in our cancer badges with the (P) crossed out. I was so relieved and happy to hear her announcement that I immediately smiled and laughed out loud. We didn't have cancer anymore! That's who Sandi is!

When I, like Jacob in Genesis 28:16, awoke from my slumber, I said, "God was in this place, and I knew it not!" When I stepped away from the puzzle, the pieces started to fit and the breathtaking picture was revealed. I realized that every time I opened up to receiving God, I was bestowed with my greatest gifts here on earth.

As I began to understand Truth, I began to distinctly remember times when I had been in my Truth during my life:

- When I was 11, I went up to my German Shepard Oliver's doghouse, took him off his leash, brought him to the garage, and held him because I somehow knew he was going to die that morning.
- Late at night after a long flight from halfway around the world, I was driving from Los Angeles to San Diego for the first time. I was tired and just trying to get to my destination when out of nowhere, in an instant, I knew I needed to move there, which I did four months later, and stayed for thirteen years.

- The moment I looked at my now husband, who at the time was just some guy I had only casually known for four days, and I knew that he would be the father of my children.
- The first time my son Daniel looked at me after he was born, I knew he knew I was his mom.
- When my son Sam was born, love and happiness overwhelmed all my senses simultaneously and filled my body to the point of bursting.
- When our Golden Retriever Jake was sick, my husband and kids were with him at the veterinarian's all morning. When I arrived at noon, he saw me and somehow found the strength to get up and walk over to me. The doctor said he was doing better, but when Jake looked into my eyes, I knew he wanted me to hold him as he passed. I walked the few feet with him back to the pen where they were keeping him, sat down, and let his head rest in my lap as he died.

Until you acknowledge Truth, take it and place it in your heart, you do not fully possess the power of your Truth. Truth is always there. Truth is God. Although overlooked, it remains constant. You may hide Truth from your mind, your words, or your actions, yet it remains… always. It takes faith to bow your head while opening your heart, and experience something unfamiliar. It takes a willingness to see what has yet to be seen, hear what has yet to be heard, and believe in what you do not yet know.

The beauty of Truth, although dismissed, degraded, and disbelieved in many ways every day for years, decades, or a lifetime, does not cease to be. It patiently sits there and waits to again be recognized. It does not judge you for overlooking it, disrespecting it, forgetting it, or calling it a lie. Truth welcomes you with love. Truth tells you that you are forgiven.

Truth sits beyond human frailty.

"And the peace of God, which passeth all understanding, shall keep your hearts and minds through Jesus Christ" Philippians 4:7

"O Lord, My God, I cried out to you, and you healed me." Psalm 30:2

The other side of knowing that the tumor would grow back when I was in the hospital is that now I know I will never get breast cancer again. I know that is my Truth. The day after Sandi announced on the shuttle that we were cancer-free, I had my end-of-treatment checkup. I was meeting with yet another oncologist. As we talked, he looked sad and helpless about my situation. It was awkward watching him calculating in his head the high odds of me getting cancer back, coupled with knowing that when triple-negative comes back, chemo really doesn't work. He also knew that if it came back it would most likely return within the next twelve months. I sat there in silence watching him play out the whole scenario in his head, reexamining the report we just spoke about, which said I still had one nodule left in my lung. He did not accept my words that lots of people have nodules in their lungs. I just looked at him, grateful that he cared enough to feel sorry, yet feeling that it was unnecessary that he do so.

As I sat there, my Truth began to rise in me. As it rose in my stomach, I sensed it. I felt timid in its presence, so I fidgeted a little until I was able to give it the space of acceptance in my heart. As I relaxed and let it move through my body, I was able to deliver my Truth to him in a natural and decisive manner. I knew he would most likely not accept my Truth but felt I needed to offer him my reassurance anyway. By offering it to him, I was honoring it within me. I embraced my quiet knowing of the sweet Truth about my cancer—not his or anyone else's truth… mine. As *my* cancer, it was mine to know about in a way his texts, studies, and other patients could never tell him. It was my Truth to know when it was gone. Gone for good, not lurking as I knew it was when they said it wasn't.

He sat *Here* at his small desk on one side of the room, knowing everything he had studied and experienced about cancer for fifteen-plus years. I sat *Over There* on the cold examining table on the other side of the room, with hair stubs, a swollen face, and flat chest, only knowing one cancer—mine—for the past ten months. How could he know that I knew something he wasn't privileged to know at that moment, my real Truth? He could not fathom that the Truth was sitting on my side of the room. I told him my Truth. "Don't worry; I'm going to be fine. I'm not going to get it back. It's okay; don't worry about me." He just looked at me with a distant pity for my naivety about cancer. I knew he felt like the oncologist who laughed at me, so sure that my tumor wouldn't grow back in a few weeks, and wanted to say, "That's not the way cancer works." I wanted to respond, "Maybe not, but that's the way *my* cancer works."

The most beautiful thing in life, when you are closest to God, is when you experience your Truth. I love finding Truth. I welcome Truth. Sitting in your Truth is one of the most complete feelings of wholeness you can ever experience. My cousin Joy told me it's called discernment when you are able to hear the Truth of God. It could be a melody. It could be a line from a movie. It could be a snowflake. It could be watching a baby being born. Truth stirs you. It swirls in the emotions of joyfulness and loving. The recognition of Truth puts a lump in your throat, makes your heart race, and brings you to the brink of tears. It casts away all illusions, giving you a moment to experience and touch the majesty of God.

He called me HERcules. I call him a healer of God.

Even though I knew my cancer was gone, the aftermath of the fire left my body in shambles. I needed to clean my physical house, so I went to a clinic in Mexico. I ate pure food and drank a lot of organic carrot and apple juice. At the clinic, I met people with cancer from all over the world. Many had stage four cancer, which meant their cancer had metastasized or spread to other parts of their body from the original site. Since they had already done many rounds of chemo, surgery, and radiation, they were now healing their immune systems so they could heal their bodies.

Even though the clinic did not care if I had Blue Cross or Blue Shield, they really *did* care about me and everyone else who went there to heal. Even though two weeks there cost less than one round of chemo here, the love and healing was miraculous. The welcome was not calculated, nor was it the same for everyone. Its only goal was to meet every part of you exactly where you were with genuine love and care. You could feel and see healing in people within a matter of days of their arrival.

The doctor in charge of healing us was the secret ingredient in everyone's transformation. Organic carrot and apple juice went a long way, but the doctor was the real elixir. He had the spirit of God in him. He met with you every day to review your progress and talk with you, and not just about cancer, but life. He believed every day and every part of it was captivating and should be received as a gift. He believed healing was as natural as the sun shining. That doctor knew the most natural act of the immune system is to heal and is activated by the most natural act of God… love.

He told me that the reason I would not die from cancer was because I didn't die from the chemo. He said he had never met anyone before who had had as much chemo as I did and lived. That's why I was not going to die; my body was strong and my spirit was alive. I also knew I was going to live—and now make sure I lived life as he did! His healing gift to me was showing me how to live fully and embrace every part of every day.

I went to the clinic in the middle of January, almost ten months to the day after I ingested my first chemo. The temperature was a relaxing seventy degrees. My mom and I sat outside in the comforting sunshine every day after breakfast with all of our new friends. We sat under luscious palm trees inside a simple yet beautiful garden courtyard, surrounded by colorful flowers and greenery. We were warmly coddled inside this garden on all four sides by white stucco buildings and painted white cement walls that made you feel protected. You could sit in this beautiful, mystical garden and feel relaxed and secure all day, every day. Even though you knew that outside those walls lay the piles of garbage, stray dogs, and hustlers of Tijuana, it didn't matter. You were safe in the garden. I sat there with people of all colors, ages, and backgrounds from all around the world. As a salesperson who could always peg everyone's position in life, I, for the first time, would not have known whose worldly titles belonged to whom if I had not been told. There was an engineer, the owner of a multi-chain restaurant business, a teacher, an owner of a technology company, a homemaker, a doctor, a lawyer, pharmacist, college students, and retirees. For the first time in my life I watched relationships that were only based on the equalizing Godliness of this place. No one judged themselves as more or *less than* anyone else. My amigos were from China, Canada, Taiwan, New York, California, Australia, Mexico, Ukraine, Illinois, and Florida.

We would all sit in the garden and share everything we knew about life, love, and God. Everyone welcomed and embraced everyone else and found ways to communicate through beautiful smiles, hugs, and language translation phone apps. Everyone interacted as equals—as more than enoughs, not *less thans*. In the safe, sunny garden, no one was sick, no one was worried. No one was giving up or fighting, only asking for what would be. Everyone was able to breathe and just be who they were… a part of God. The garden showed me the physical portrait of *Over There*. It was a safe place where everyone could stand in their moment and take in life as it was given and meant to be, only with pure love. Those two weeks showed me that peace like that is possible *Here* for a lifetime, the rest of my lifetime. We really do have the ability to be on earth as we are in heaven. I wish everyone in the world would be able to experience humanity from the perspective of those people I sat with who were possibly leaving it. People who made their peace with their humanness and embraced their holiness. People who could sit with God in this world for the remainder of their time *Here* and be in beautiful peace. Watching and being with people who have every reason to fall apart yet sit in pure peace… it is the miracle of seeing God.

Satan is usually pictured in a red suit in cartoons, sitting on someone's shoulder and telling them to do the wrong thing. Although I know that the devil is not a cartoon character, I do think the cartoonists' depiction of him is more accurate than most of us think. The devil's negative whisper is a voice in your mind that casts darkness over the light of your good thoughts, not just your deeds and actions but your outlook and ideas.

After I returned from Mexico and was beginning to get stronger, I began having vivid dreams. While I'm asleep, I am often aware of my dreams and I watch them as if they are a show on television. During this one particular dream, I was watching two young girls talking about me and overheard them saying something vague about being surprised about me because I looked so good. My mind immediately thought they must be talking about me getting sick again. That thought was not part of the dream. It came from my mind as I was watching the dream. I then started to feel devastated, thinking the dream was telling me I was going to die. That's when I once again heard the calm female voice of God. She interrupted my fearful thoughts and spoke from a firm, solid, yet loving stance on my behalf, and in a way that everyone understood that her words would be followed. She was not directing her decree at me, though; she was talking to where the negative thoughts came from, and she said, "Oh, no, you are not doing that to her." I knew she was not talking to me, as I was just watching and hearing the girls talking in the dream when I heard the thoughts outside of the dream. The negative thoughts that started the spiral of fear came from outside of what I was watching and hearing in my dream. It was like there were three of us involved in the conversation: me, as the observer of the dream; the fearful thoughts; and the female voice. The female voice was standing up for me as I watched the dream and became scared by the thoughts that made me think this dream was showing me that I was going to die. She was clearly talking to the place where the fearful thoughts arose and telling it that it was not going to do that to me. She was talking to the place in my mind that creates negativity, fear, and doom; the place of the devil I had heard about so many times. I now know that one aspect of the devil everyone fears resides in the subconscious negative part of my mind that comes up with thoughts that cause fear and pain.

After that night when I was awake and fearful thoughts like that would again surface, I would always remember the female voice's calm and sure words. I would remember how the woman's voice defended me against that exact same kind of thoughts in my dream, and I would use her words during the day: "Oh, no, you're not going to do that to me." I learned that, even if my heart was with God and knew the fact that I was not going to get cancer again, my subconscious negative mind would still try to convince me otherwise. However, I also knew that, with God on my side, the devil in my mind could cause a racket but not a revolution.

That is the infinite power of God. God always trumps anything not of God! It became much easier to stop listening to my mind's false thoughts, which tried to convince me that its malicious fear was necessary to keep me safe, when I realized that those thoughts were coming from something trying to deceive and hurt me. Now, every time my mind starts being negative, I know that non-sense is not coming from me or God. Today, the only question I have to ask myself about negative thoughts is, "Do I want to sit with this lie and feel like hell or do I want to stand in my Truth and feel peace with the heavenly voice of God?"

When I stood by the fire, it burned parts of me that meant too much. So I stepped away, finding man's safety, which turned out to be my cross. Then ever after came. Once I let go, like a firefly, I began to instinctually light up, carrying the flame. With the heat of hallowedness, I was able to move in, out, and through. When I was without fear, I learned what I already knew. The fire healed my heart's pain. As I stepped out and stood again by the fire, I remembered the fear—but not of the flames, just of the years in refrain. So I sat back upon a solid rock and, from the warmth, I began to see the sacredness of the flames in me. It was then I found the unfolding of the Truth that had been so distorted in my youth. I want to show others the sacredness of the flames. I want them to rise and call God by His name. I want them to know that they can find their sacredness as it has always remained, but only if they are willing to fly with and within the flames.

How does living in your Truth work? I struggled with this. I didn't know what my life would be like if I lived from the Truth of God versus what I had done in the past—only living through my mind. I didn't know how to be with God in the world of everyday life, with deadlines, bills, chores, and traffic. I was gaining my physical strength and my ability to think again. I knew I was being pulled back like a nail to the magnet of my old world. The thought was alluring; just putting the whole debacle of the last sixteen months behind me and getting back to the big bad business of being me, chasing more money, more success, and letting my ego hold my "survivorship" as its prize.

I couldn't do it. I could not hit the *play* button. The red carpet was rolled out for my arrival. *Wait… what… WHAT?* I did not want to go back to what I longed for and had pressed my face up against the window begging for, because the grass was actually greener *Over There.* I could not let go of my connection to God. I relished the feeling of being in a safe, quiet car. I could no longer bear the speed and noise of the shiny racecar. The sound of the racing engine and swirling of the air was now too loud, and it made me uncomfortable. I knew I really wanted to stay in the quiet and peaceful safety of God.

That summer I made the decision to trade in my old life and search out something new. Did I go to a religious retreat or an ashram? No. I went to the front porch of our new house. Well, it was almost a hundred years new and had this great enclosed front porch lined all around with old wooden windows. I swept out the leaves that had blown in there and scrubbed it good, washing off all of the old dirt and dust. The newly washed, sturdy wood floor now had a bit of a shine—but more importantly it held a cozy loveseat where I could sit to look outside at the world. I would open all the windows so the fresh air could flow through. I would sit there and look out at the abundant greenery, beautifully framed by the white window trim and pastel yellow of the walls. I would sit and watch the world pass through.

I would drift out there every day, often a couple of times a day. I would stare off, drifting back to the place *Over There*; a place that I had not known existed just months earlier. I loved the time that I could slip away from *Here* to be *Over There* and be with God. While I sat there, I also tried to remember what I had learned in the past sixteen months. I knew I was different but was not sure what had happened. I wanted to piece it all together to understand what I had learned about God and myself.

I tried to write down what I had remembered from along the way, but I had to stop because it was still too hot to hold. Many of the chapters of this book were written in a two-week period out on that porch, but I had to lay them down for another four months because I needed the space to accept them in order to hold them. I talked to trusted friends about what some called my Dark Night of the Soul. I kept asking God to show me how to do this. I told Him I wanted to live in the world differently but did not know how.

In every single beautiful moment, you can make a new choice to move back to the other side of you, the Truth of you, the holiness of you, and into the tranquil peace of God's love. Even though I can now freely move back and forth, I still sometimes forget about Over There during the day. The important thing is that I

now know there is always another choice. There always was—I just need to remember it.

I began to notice that I was experiencing the world differently. I went back to doing all the things I had always done, but now somehow everything had changed. For the first time making a sandwich was *just making a sandwich.* I wasn't on a conference call with the mute button on, or thinking about something else that this sandwich-making was keeping me from doing, or hoping to finish faster so I could check it off my to-do list. I was simply and beautifully now *just making a sandwich.* I was not just physically making that sandwich, but my mind and heart were there with me as I made those sandwiches, and the whole experienced changed.

Time also changed when I started making sandwiches that way—and doing everything that way. Time became timeless and my days felt much fuller and seemed to last much longer because I was savoring every moment and no longer squeezing the life out of them. I was no longer squandering my place in the world, but wholly residing in it. That's how I found my way back into this world, but now with God: making sandwiches every day for my sons, and making organic carrot and apple juice for me. Being with my kids and having lunch. Not taking a break from anything to have lunch but being in the wholeness of my day and sitting down with my kids and eating lunch. No thought of what I had been doing before or what I would be doing next. The only thing that mattered at lunch was being there shooing away the bees, feeling the sun, laughing, and watching the joy on my kids' faces as they had lunch with their mom. When I first begged for my life and cried to be saved from cancer, I did so mainly to remain physically here and raise my kids. However, it turns out I received much more than that. I am now *wholly* here to raise my children, not just physically but to have them experience all of me. My wholeness and knowing of life and Truth can show them how to find theirs. To create a world where peace prevails, we must first find it within ourselves. There is no greater gift we can bestow upon our children than showing them our reflection of peace so that they can see their Truth.

At the close of every day, I would turn off the television and all the lights in the living room just to sit still for fifteen minutes in the quietness the world permitted after the rest of the house went to sleep. It was easy peace and one of the best parts of my day. I would thank God for getting me to this place of peace and for healing my body. I would thank Him for never judging me and for only offering His endless loving patience. I would then go to sleep not needing to sigh that it all remained intact—because it always was. I would drift into sleep and learn things in my dreams about God, about moving deeper *Over There*, and finding ways to make peace with what had happened *Here*. I would again hear my familiar female voice of God in my dreams.

Putting my life down in words has allowed me to find the remarkable wisdom from the people and events I met along the way. I now truly appreciate the story of The Wizard of Oz. Chemo required me to find enough courage to let go and reach for something greater than Here. Others' compassion and prayers showed me the power of love to fix my broken heart. Falling over and over helped me remember what I had forgotten. And everything combined led me to find my Truth in Almighty God and to live life for the first time in peace. I no longer needed to be the big, boisterous Wizard of Oz character who was larger than life, trying to be more. The woman behind the curtain has learned she always was more than enough just as she was. She was a part of God, who is everything.

During the transition to my new life, I wasn't really sure whom I was anymore. I would still get lost between *Here* and *Over There.* I felt fragile. For someone who never felt anything other than invincible as I held up my *more than* shield, fragile made me feel tentative about my movements through the world. Now, after laying down my thunderous *more than* shield, I had to learn how to feel comfortable holding my newfound quiet and peaceful strength given by God.

I would also feel humbled. Not in the sense of feeling *less than* but humbled in awe of the easy peace and stillness I now had. I loved it but didn't quite know what to do with it. I also didn't know what to do when I would experience a rush of love that would arrive from *Over There* that would reverberate through my heart. It was a feeling I had never known. It was all remarkable yet confusing to me; I did not know it was possible to feel such strength and security coming from a place of stillness, peace, love, and light.

Even with all of my insides fumbling around, I was again able to be doing "normal life" things. One Saturday I dropped my sons off at a birthday party in Fargo and decided to spend the next hour and a half looking for some new clothes. I walked into the department store on a tight timeline and headed back to the clothing section. As I was walking forward toward the dresses, I suddenly decided to make a right turn, as I was being drawn to the jewelry section. I was mad at myself for not following my plan, knowing I didn't have a lot of time, but I kept heading there anyway.

Since having kids, I did not wear a lot of jewelry unless I was on a business trip. I usually only wore my wedding ring. We were also now on a tight budget since my brain wasn't really operating like it used to and I wasn't sure if I would be able to continue working. I went over there anyway, telling myself I would just take a quick look. Who knows; something might be on sale. I thought I would see if they had any heart necklaces since my heart was now so full of joy. The sales associate put a heart charm I had picked out onto a silver chain. The charm did not look quite right once I tried it on, so I went to the other side of the counter to see if there were any other hearts that might look better. Over there I saw a silver cross pendant with a diamond in the middle of it. I never thought that I would be a person who advertised her belief in God. I knew that was taboo in the business world—and, frankly, previously in my personal world. I did not want to wear a cross around my neck, inviting people's judgments of me. For crying out loud, I still hadn't read the Bible and didn't even go to church most Sundays—how could I wear a cross necklace? Since I would not stop looking at it, the sales associate suggested I try it on. I was still unsure about doing so but gave in anyway. Once I put it on and looked at it in the mirror, I knew I could not take it off. I was supposed to wear it. The day I tried the cross necklace on and knew it fit, I heard my Truth, and I now wear it every day. As I now look at it around my neck, I again feel the humbleness and strength of easy peace and joy given to me by God.

When I later shared this story with someone, I was told that the cross symbolizes heaven; spirituality, and earth; physical experience, integrated within the human being, bringing wholeness.

I also learned that Carl Jung, a psychotherapist called the Father of Psychology, reviewed thousands of cases that he had overseen, and one common theme consistently occurred prior to a patient's healing: patients who were ultimately and permanently healed all shared the same image of the universal symbol of a circle with a cross. The manifestation of this image could have taken place in their thoughts, dreams, drawings, or other physical forms. This symbolism was an indication that the individual was again rebalancing their mental and physical health and returning to their spiritual center.

Buying this cross was not just a symbol of my healing through my new wholeness, balance, and spirituality. It was the first time since I found God that I was able to speak to the world about my knowing of Him. I was not yet ready to use my voice, but for the first time, I was not afraid to show that I was with Him.

The remains of cancer treatment allow me to know that being human is a state of vulnerability. Man's vulnerability cannot be relieved, thus eliminating his fear, through any device man has created. Everyone has fear when they are without God.

My hair at sixteen months after chemo is now back to my normal bob cut. It has its bounce back. Everyone thinks I am back to my old self, but what only my husband and kids see is that I still have half chemo hair. My hair is half Bozo the Clown, crazy-chemoed, dried-out, curly hair, and the newer half is full, straight, soft, bouncy hair. It's okay that it is still half crazy. I am still human after all. What is most beautiful now is that I can smooth out the falseness of my old chemoed hair into the softness of my new hair. I can be an erroneous human but be tempered by the gentleness of the hand of God. I talk a lot about my fear during cancer, but the truth is I was afraid every day before that too. It just had a different label back then: being alone without God and not being good enough.

I can still be tough, and know that the part of me that has had plenty of practice speaking loudly, while swinging the powerful gavel of judgment against myself and others, is still there. It is no longer a constant state of mind though. Now when it happens, it no longer feels comfortable. I am no longer numb to the pain that I inflict on others and myself. I am more aware of that pain, which was always ricocheting back to me, and it stings me awake again. I have learned how to move out of my *less than* thinking, leaving me the openness to find my way back to peace. I am here on this earth and I am walking this planet in human form. That is the physical truth. I always got that. What I somehow lost along the way was that I am also a part of God in human form, walking on this planet. I am other than my reflection in the mirror. I am the Truth beyond what can be seen with my human eyes.

Shoes that I used to wear so comfortably. Shoes that helped me project to the world what I thought it wanted to see. Shoes that worked with the hem of my pants, allowing them to hang exacting to the floor, now hurt. Shoes that once seemed comfortable now created pain. My foot is the same size on the outside, but the inside workings of my foot have changed.

The Taxol chemo left lasting nerve damage in my last three toes on both of my feet. They always have numbness and tingling, like when a body part goes to sleep, especially the baby toe on my right foot. Both of the balls-of-my feet are also numb, and when I walk it feels like there is a piece of cardboard superglued to my skin. When I'm inside my house, I usually do not wear shoes, and my foot pain is bearable. To go outside, I now have to buy wide-width shoes, not because my feet are wider but now their ability to remain in the confined space that most shoes provide can begin a cascade of nerve pain. It leads right up the center of my feet, causing them to feel like they are on fire. So when I pick my shoes, I have to choose carefully now, knowing that most of them will not fit right. I also have to walk more consciously. When I have to wear shoes that no longer fit right, I have to decide wisely where I'm going, on what type of surface I will walk, how much pressure I will put into each step, and for how long I will wear them.

My feet have become a metaphor for my life after cancer. They acknowledge the journey that brought me here today had to be walked one step at a time. They also serve as a reminder of what happens when you deny your Truth and keep believing that something outside of you is going to save you. But, most importantly, the blessing of my feet is that they are a physical reminder that I no longer want to walk painfully through life without God as I did before. I know now that I have to be mindful of the steps I choose to take and what shoes I choose to walk in.

PART 7

Beautiful Truth

"God is the perfect poet." – Robert Browning

That's why I would hear the whispers along the way, saying that it was going to be okay. It always was.

I did not find all of my Truth at once; that's just not how it worked for me. My knowing of God has been like the old car I used to drive in high school with a clogged carburetor. It was hard to start, hard to move forward, and stalled a lot. I soon learned I could put an object like a screwdriver in the carburetor to prop it open while I was starting the car so enough air could make it through and allow the engine to run. Sometimes I would get my car on the road chugging forward a bit and then it would shut down again. Once I learned how to clean out the debris so the air could continually flow in, I no longer had to constantly lift the hood and find something to prop open the carburetor for fresh air. The car then ran better and my life became easier.

My faith and knowing of God, although not built with speed, was formed securely, upon a very solid foundation. The time it took was necessary because it takes time to instill your soul's memory in your heart. In the beginning, I didn't even know there was another part of this life. I had no idea that *Over There* was another place that sat right behind my heart. Once you find *Over There*, your Truth in God, you know time is really timeless.

God has no deadline for us to remember *Over There*. He waits with only loving patience, allowing us the choice to remember. He is always reminding us of this place through people, situations, and love. All we have to do is look and hear what is coming from behind our hearts to remember what we have forgotten. Remembering brings us His love and peace. God is overjoyed when we find Him again. He welcomes you back without judgment and with open arms that hold more love than you have ever known.

Always know that your choice for life and Truth is always just one more choice away. You can change your mind and make a new choice in any instant. Each wrong choice allows you a new opportunity to discover the right choice. I cannot sit here today and say that if I had made different choices I would have been better or worse off than the way it unfolded. There was only ever one choice for me and for everyone: returning home to God either while you are still in your body or not. There are many paths that lead there. The trail I walked was not comfortable or glamorous; it was simply my choice. I believe that whatever you choose, God is with you. You can hold His hand or pretend He's not there. You can sit in a quiet room and find peace or burn out your bone marrow and hold your feet to the fire. I did the latter.

The business of being human is messy. My story was painfully messy. Every time I read it, I think, *Seriously, how could you continue such a destructive pattern of thinking over and over?* It was easier than it looked. Humans tend to do what they always have done in terms of how they think and consequently how they behave. What's hard is getting out of your long-standing patterns because that requires you to slog through the mess they sit in. It takes time and is not a straight path. Some people have a miraculous awakening in an instant that changes everything. The rest of us have to do the work to make our new choices happen while we are still running into walls and beating ourselves up along the way. The good news is, God does not give you points based on style, neatness, or lack of pain. God rewards everyone with the same peace just for making it *Over There.*

By the end of my unexpected and chaotic journey, I did make changes; pretty big ones. They were not neatly labeled as they are written about here. They didn't happen in an orderly procession. Lessons were taught and retaught to me many times before they were understood. Insights that you thought would have come first came later, and many changes happened without my full awareness of how or why. And I never really pieced it all together until I wrote this book. So I'm telling you that no matter how many times you get lost on your journey and how many times you circle around where you want to be, but can't find the right road, or miss the signs, it's okay. The right roads and signs are still there. Just take a breath, fill up your tank and keep going. Keep your mind clear in the knowing that you are headed to the destination of Truth.

It doesn't matter how you get there. It just matters that you keep asking God to show you the way. I was so deep in the thicket of the maze that I had no idea what was happening or how it was happening. I didn't even know where my new path was taking me, or if I was going to get to what would save me. Even after finding God, I didn't know if I had found what would change my life's course. I just kept searching for new ways to live while building a deeper relationship with God. I had no idea that my answers were in God; it took me a while to understand how His love worked. But that's okay because I had His grace with me even before I remembered mine. When I learned to trust in God and silence my mind, I could then hold God's hand. Once I could do that, I was free. So don't get wrapped up in the details of your story as it unfolds; keep moving forward, reaching for and then holding the hand of the God, who has written it. Know where you want to end up. Know that you are seeking the Truth of yourself. Know that is God.

Anyone who wants to find God only needs to seek Him with a completely open and loving mind and heart. He is not hidden. Anyone who comes from a pure and honest place of wanting to know God, with genuine openness and love in their heart to the possibility, will come to know God. Even before someone again chooses to find and then remember God, they should know that they are still a part of Him every day. That makes me happy. No one is left out. Everyone is in.

Those who seek and find God, those in the process, and those who do not want to are all children of the same almighty God. The only difference is on this side of the equation. Those who know and accept God's love have a peace that those who don't know him can't conceive. That doesn't make those who know Him better or more *of God*, just more at peace. But that's okay; everyone is free to be with God or not. It is a choice, after all. God loves you either way.

If you are now sick and think making a new choice to live through God could help your healing, it's important to also include other care your healing formula. When I was searching for what I needed to save my life, I used both traditional and non-traditional avenues of treatment. Even though ultimately my greatest healing came from healing my heart, living with God, I knew my sick body needed to be attended to as well. I included all possibilities of healing in order to save my life, healing my mind, soul, *and* body.

Some people will choose chemo, as I did. Would that be my choice again? I used to say no, but now I would not rewrite my past. My feet might, but I will not. Did chemo set back my immune system and physical healing? Yes. Did it take me to the depths of despair and the brink of death which allowed me to heal my mind? Yes. Never judge yourself or others by what choices are made when someone is so deep in the storm. You never know why until it is revealed. You only need to know that it is as it should be. When you have peace in your heart, you will know what the right choices are for your healing.

Nine months before writing this book, I could not see the screen on my television due to the nerve damage chemo inflicted on my eyes. Eight months prior, I had both of my breasts removed, one with a tumor that was still more than half its original size after six months of chemotherapy. One month later, I could not lift my arm or feel any part of my upper arm from the mastectomy. Six months before using my computer to write this book, I was unable to count out the change from my purse when I was trying to pay for groceries because my brain was still too heavily under the influence of chemo. Five months prior, I could not walk, only shuffle after 8:00 p.m. at night, due to the nerve damage in my feet. Four months before writing this book, I was not able to read more than three pages of a book before I had to take a nap, because it tired my brain. For all the damage to my physical state, I knew that the body is miraculous and all it ever wants to do is heal—and mine for the most part has. The body will never stop trying to heal; it has the miracle of healing always. I knew it was up to me to change my mind so I could open my heart and allow all possible healing in.

As my heart was healing, the distance between me and my holiness was easier to cross making it more comfortable to feel and hear the voice of God. I had no idea He was inside of me. I thought God was down the street at the pizza shop or up in the clouds somewhere. The first time I realized that I could feel Him and His love beamed through my healing heart, I cried. I began to remember what I had lost. Now that I know that God is inside me, I can freely dash back and forth between my human life and the space of God in an instant, feeling worthy enough to do so without any reason except to hang out in the peace of God. I carry Him in my heart *Here* and find His love, safety, and peace *Over There.*

Like my journey, my changes were not perfect or complete but were enough to heal me. You don't have to be perfect to heal; you have to relieve enough of the stress your mind puts in your body to free up enough energy for your immune system to heal you. My changes lifted the constant stress of the world I had created inside of my mind that always told me that God was not there, and that I had to do more and be better so that I would not be rejected. These changes were enough… not everything, but enough for me to take a deep breath and feel the stress of my old way of living disappear. Enough to let me live through God's eternal life and feel peace. Enough to cure my cancer. I don't know what you need to do to heal, or even if healing is the part of the covenant you have made with God for this life. Those Truths are only for you to know. However, I do know that your negative mind's false beliefs have a powerful effect on your body and it wants to keep you from God's healing love.

The irony of my writing a book about God is not lost on me. If you had asked me before cancer if I would have written a paragraph about God, I would have given you a *believer/non-believer* side glance and laughed out loud, saying I would be the last person to tell anyone about God.

This book started only as a personal journal to compile the thoughts and events that I felt compelled to write down shortly after my treatment was over. A few months later, I wanted to piece everything together that had happened to me, to understand why I was now so different than before I had cancer. I then started filling in the rest of the story with my other memories. Everything in my head was still tangled and out of order. I wrote whatever came up in my mind, regardless of the timeline. I just kept writing until it all came out. Sometimes what I wrote overwhelmed me and I needed to set it aside. Other times I read and reread my words, unable to set them down and move on because they so honestly and beautifully spoke of God. I then took the jumble of emotions and events and placed them in chronological order as best I could, so I could move through the experience from start to finish and understand what had happened to save my life *and* completely change my life.

Once I started reading about the people, events, and circumstances of my cancer journey, the meanings became self-evident. What occurred as I began to understand what really happened was the finding of the spectacular unflinching Truth of God. As I saw the hand of God in everything, it took my breath away. I couldn't believe how everything fit together and made perfect sense in the light of Truth. I was finally putting my beautiful picture together that I had wanted for so long. I had no idea that it would be found through cancer and God. It took piecing all the fireworks together to understand the grandness of the finale. Maybe that's why He saved me: so a *believer/non-believer* could share with others the beautiful Truth of God.

I no longer think I am a singular being, a standalone unit. I am part of God, which encompasses all the love and all the knowing in the Universe. That's what makes the whole experience of cancer so trite and the whole experience of finding God so humbling. You think you are this little separate *less than, Here*, when you are really a part of the immenseness and greatness of *Over There*. It rewrites the story of the *less than* ugly duckling. Now God's duckling already knows it is more than enough and loved by the divine, understanding that its destiny is exquisitely breathtaking and beautifully created, guided, and preordained by what is both seen and unseen.

I am now grateful that I got cancer and did not have a heart attack. Cancer was the right cure for my heart that was constantly under attack by my mind. Cancer allowed me the time to sit in the hurt I had allowed into my heart and find my breath from God, allowing me to change my mind. Once I discovered how to still my mind and learned how to let everything pass through my Truth, my heart could release all the pain and open up, becoming light and steady. I was always aware of my heart straining, even before cancer, from walking up the stairs or when I flinched from everyday life's shrapnel. It was wounded and heavy. I know I was right; cancer was not going to take me out—my heart was. I just didn't know how. Today I seldom think about my heart. It is now quiet, steady, and healed. It is calm and peaceful because it is with God.

I no longer sit righteously between religion and spirituality. I now sit there humbly and openly accepting of what each offers to help me move across my bridge to God. I can find my way to the Truth and light of God through Jesus' teachings. I have found my way to the place of God through peaceful walks in the woods. I can cross over through the beautiful processions and rituals of religion, or simply putting my hand on my heart and feeling it beat. I can also sit comfortably in the warm sunshine on my front porch and bask in the glory of God. When I'm with God and experience His eternal love of me so far beyond what my humanness can create I'm at peace and it does not matter through which crossing I arrive.

My learning and my love of God is deep but not yet wide. I found the essential truths of God that set me free and allowed me to enter my Truth and live in the peace of God. The way I found Him, and how I truly came to be with Him was through my heart, not my mind. I have only experienced unfaltering love and acceptance from God, wrapped up in the feeling of eternal peace. He is the endless part of me and I reside within Him. I am grateful and blessed to know enough of God to be with Him every day. I don't profess to *know everything* about God. But I do confess to *knowing* Him and receiving life through him. I don't proclaim to understand everything that is contained in the air I breathe, but I do know how to accept with gratitude the life I receive through it. I can tell you that I love God from a profound and devoted place. I feel and live in His grace and love. I can say that words will never adequately express the experience of God.

I wish that the knowing and relationship I have with God could be experienced by everyone, because it makes life much more alive, yet peaceful, and every moment a breathtaking occasion. God never tried to change my mind about Him. His love and complete acceptance allowed me to escape the false beliefs of my mind that kept me from Him. He patiently waited for me behind my heart until I opened it up to the possibility of being with Him and hearing His voice.

Know that God is waiting for you too—*Over There* behind your heart. I promise!

The LORD is my shepherd; I shall not want.

He maketh me lie down in green pastures: he leadeth me beside still waters.

He restoreth my soul: he leadeth me in the paths of righteousness for his name's sake. Yea, though I walk through the valley of the shadow of death, I will fear no evil: for thou art with me; thy rod and thy staff they comfort me.

Thou preparest a table before me in the presence of mine enemies: though anointest my head with oil; my cup runneth over.

Surely goodness and mercy shall follow me all the days of my life: and I will dwell in the house of the LORD for ever. Psalm 23

Made in the USA
Las Vegas, NV
28 January 2024